[美国] 克里斯蒂安·W. 麦克米伦 著　李超群 译

牛津通识读本·

大流行病

Pandemics

A Very Short Introduction

译林出版社

图书在版编目（CIP）数据

　　大流行病 ／（美）克里斯蒂安·W. 麦克米伦著；李超群译.
—南京：译林出版社，2022.6
　　（牛津通识读本）
　　书名原文：Pandemics: A Very Short Introduction
　　ISBN 978-7-5447-8613-3

　　Ⅰ.①大… 　Ⅱ.①克…②李… 　Ⅲ.①流行病学－研究
Ⅳ.①R18

中国版本图书馆 CIP 数据核字（2022）第 057358 号

著作权合同登记号　图字：10-2020-086 号

大流行病　[美国] 克里斯蒂安·W. 麦克米伦／著　李超群／译

责任编辑　许　丹
装帧设计　景秋萍
校　　对　王　敏
责任印制　董　虎

原文出版　Oxford University Press, 2016
出版发行　译林出版社
地　　址　南京市湖南路 1 号 A 楼
邮　　箱　yilin@yilin.com
网　　址　www.yilin.com
市场热线　025-86633278
排　　版　南京展望文化发展有限公司
印　　刷　江苏扬中印刷有限公司
开　　本　890 毫米 ×1260 毫米　1/32
印　　张　9.125
插　　页　4
版　　次　2022 年 6 月第 1 版
印　　次　2022 年 6 月第 1 次印刷
书　　号　ISBN 978-7-5447-8613-3
定　　价　39.00 元

序　言

张大庆

　　作为一本试图从宏观层面勾勒瘟疫与人类历史演进的通识读本，本书选取了鼠疫、天花、疟疾、霍乱、结核、流感和艾滋病等七种主要的大流行病，讲述了每种疾病的生物学特性及其如何导致了传染病的大流行。作者将科学的解释与历史文化分析巧妙结合，还论及当代的流行病，如新发传染病埃博拉出血热、寨卡热以及禽流感等。

　　著名历史学家麦克尼尔曾指出，在人类历史的进程中，传染病一直都扮演着关键性的角色。传染病是微生物与人类相互作用的结果。微生物是地球上最古老的生命之一，也伴随着人类的进化与大流行病的肆虐。它不仅严重地危及人类的生命，而且会造成人们的恐慌心理，影响社会经济和国际贸易。这次"新冠肺炎"的暴发再次证明，流行病不仅可以重塑人类的历史，同时，人类的行为也在影响着流行病的进程与转归。

　　回顾人类与微生物两者之间的关系和共同演化的历程，我们发现，自人类社会早期开始，瘟疫就是影响人类文化的关键因素。人类在狩猎和采集活动中，因食用动物或与动物接触而被感染，导致许多人兽共患病，如旋毛虫病、非洲睡眠病、兔热病、疟疾、血吸虫病以及钩端螺旋体病等；此外，还有一些是与人类共同进化的微生物引起的疾病，如肠道寄生虫、体虱、沙门氏菌及密螺旋体所致的雅司病和梅毒。大约在公元前500年前后，伴随古老文明中心的发展，天花、白喉、流感、水痘、流行性腮腺炎等传染病迅速地在人类之间传播。传染病的流行不仅危及个人的健康和生命，同时也影响到人类历史的发展进程。古希腊由盛转衰、古罗马帝国的瓦解与流行病的肆虐不无关系。从某种意义上说，人类文明史就是一部不断与瘟疫抗争的历史。

1960年代以后，在西方发达国家，大多数传染病已经基本被消灭，剩下的部分也可以通过免疫和抗生素得到控制，医学界转向攻克心脑血管疾病、恶性肿瘤以及其他慢性退行性病变。然而，在20世纪末，人们惊讶地发现，传染病依然还在危害人类的健康，人类与传染病的斗争尚未结束。在世界卫生组织发表的危害人类健康最严重的48种疾病中，传染病和寄生虫病占40种，发病人数占病人总数的85%。传染病依然是公共卫生不发达地区的主要问题。这次"新冠肺炎"的暴发，使人们再次清醒地认识到，人类同传染病的斗争远没有结束，任何忽视传染病控制的观点都是十分有害的。

传染病的全球化蔓延以及检疫防疫的全球化进程并非一个新问题。随着人类的迁移、贸易和殖民活动，"微生物一体化"导致了疾病尤其是传染病的全球性扩散。为了应付大流行病的肆虐，从19世纪末至20世纪中期，人们创建了许多与公共卫生有关的国际组织与机构，对大流行病的控制转向国际化行动。20

世纪初建立的国际联盟卫生组织在控制流行病蔓延、加强国际疫情通报以及协助许多国家建立公共卫生和防疫体系方面发挥了重要作用。此外，洛克菲勒基金会、国际抗结核病联盟等非政府组织也促进了国际卫生合作。第二次世界大战以后，世界卫生组织成为处理当代全球疾病控制和公共卫生问题最具影响力的组织。它展开了一系列控制疾病的全球行动：如根除天花计划，根除疟疾计划，根除麻疹、百日咳、脊髓灰质炎计划，消灭麻风、麦地那龙线虫病计划等。1958年，第11届世界卫生大会通过了根除天花决议，经过20年的艰苦努力，人类终于在1979年彻底地消灭了天花。世界卫生组织发起的根除麻疹、百日咳、脊髓灰质炎计划也基本上获得了成功。

在本书中，作者还讨论了国家在应对传染病流行时所采取的重要措施，如检疫、隔离、旅行限制和其他形式的社会管控。虽然我们已经拥有了疫苗、抗生素、化学药物等，能够有效地控制许多传染病，但在许多发展中国家一些传染病仍然具有破坏性。通过评估贫穷和疾病以及流行病地理分布之间的关系，麦克米伦就全球各国政府必须从过去的经验中吸取教训，并积极合作预防未来任何传染病的流行提出了建议。

毫无疑问，在与瘟疫的较量中，人类已经获得了巨大的胜利。但是新的致命传染病还会不时地出现，例如艾滋病、埃博拉出血热、拉沙热、马尔堡病、裂谷热、SARS以及最近暴发的COVID-19等。面对传染病，我们要有"预防胜过治疗"的理念，要提高个人的卫生意识，采取健康的生活方式，提高免疫力。总的来说，尽管我们依然会对突发的传染病产生恐慌，人类对于不断出现的传染病还有待深入认识，甚至不得不接受将与传染病长期共存的现实，但是我们也应该看到当代科学技术的发展、人类社会的发展已为我们应对传染病提供了丰富的手段。我们相信依靠科学，依靠人类的聪明才智和团结友爱的精神，我们可以从容地面对各类传染病的挑战，不断提升人类健康的水平。

大流行病

献给奥林、玛雅、斯蒂芬妮

目 录

致　谢

　　几年前，我和牛津大学的南希·托夫见面讨论合作事项。当时我正在写一本关于结核病的书。写书的过程中我对其他流行病也产生了兴趣。南希发现在"牛津通识读本"中，规模性流行病或大流行病主题仍是空白，这让我们都感到有些意外。或许我可以试一试？在南希的帮助下，我完成了这本书的创作。谢谢你，南希。牛津大学的埃尔达·格拉纳塔不厌其烦地回答了我提出的无数个问题。因为有了她，整个过程都很愉快。感谢选修了我所开的"流行病、大流行病及其历史"课程的学生们，在他们不知情的情况下，我在课堂上讲述了书中的内容并听取了他们的反馈。本书建立在许多前辈历史学家的辛勤研究之上，他们致力于发掘疾病在人类历史中的重要地位。在此向他们致以衷心的感谢。最后，一如既往地，我最想感谢我亲爱的妻子斯蒂芬妮和我们的孩子玛雅与奥林。

引　言

本书旨在介绍规模性流行病（epidemics）和大流行病（pandemics）的深远历史，并说明当今人们应对这些疾病的主要措施深受过往的影响。这看似不值一提，实际上却很重要。人们往往只有在重新遭遇当代流行病时才会回望历史，如此曾经的模式在不经意间一再重演。

规模性流行病和大流行病指的是什么？通常认为特定时间内，发病率突然大面积升高的疾病，即可被称为规模性流行病。大流行病可以被理解为超大规模的流行病。2014年的埃博拉疫情完全称得上是一次规模性流行病——甚至可以算得上大流行病。1918年夺去5 000万人性命的流感则是一次大流行病。

规模性流行病和大流行病往往被看作各种事件。事情发生了，然后又结束了。不过，如果我们这样看待流行病，那艾滋病能不能被称为大流行病？结核呢？还有疟疾呢？大流行病可以是散发事件或者是我称为持续流行的疾病。结核、疟疾和艾滋病，这些影响全球许多国家和地区，并且每年造成几百万人死亡

1

1 的疾病都是长期存在的大流行病。

2009年H1N1甲型流感期间，世界卫生组织和其他机构所使用的大流行病的定义引发了争议。在美国国立卫生研究院下属的过敏和传染性疾病研究所，有几位传染病学专家提出了一套宽泛的标准，来辅助定义大流行病。他们提出其必须满足八个条件：影响地域广阔、疾病具有流动性、感染率高而且发病迅速、群体免疫少见、属于新发疾病、可以间接传染、可以接触传染、病情严重。看起来似乎结核、艾滋病和疟疾都不是新出现的疾病，但它们的表现会有所不同。有些地方结核感染情况恶化，有些地方出现好转；广泛耐药性结核出现——结核又成了一种全新的病。每个特定的历史背景都是全新的。1950年代，世界卫生组织努力消灭疟疾时，它表现出了新的特性；1970年代和1980年代，世界银行在世界卫生领域发挥重要作用时，疟疾又有了变化。艾滋病也是如此。随着时代变迁，艾滋病的内涵经历了深刻的变化，它拥有了许多新的身份，每个身份都和历史相关：从死亡判决到慢性可控性疾病，从同性恋疾病到异性恋也会染上的疾病。

规模性流行病和大流行病的历史有一些共同的主题。19世纪末，实验室的重大发现使得人们对疾病的认识发生重要改变，这些发明引领我们进入持续至今的现代医疗时代。法国的路易斯·巴斯德所开创的，以及德国的罗伯特·科赫所传承的学说改变了疾病成因解释纷繁的状况，此后疾病的病因都只有一个解释，这一变革的影响怎样强调也不为过。细菌感染导致结核等疾病这一发现意味着延续了百年的病因说不复存在，医学科学首次能确定一种疾病的病因。人们或能真正治愈疾病。结核杆菌和鼠疫杆菌的发现使得开发和提出有效的治疗方法和预防措施成为可能。但实验室变革也催生了对生物医学能根除感染性疾病的过度信心，使得人们形成了一种信念，即要达成这一目标更多地是靠杀灭病菌，而不是改善会引发疾病的社会环境。

这引出了另外两个主题：贫穷和疾病的关系、规模性流行病和大流行病的地域特征。本书中讨论的所有疾病尽管都可以在现代医疗条件下（不同程度地）得到控制，却都受社会状况的影响。也就是说，霍乱一个多世纪前就在美国消失无踪而至今仍存在于许多发展中国家，艾滋病在撒哈拉以南的非洲地区有着不成比例的高感染率，1720年法国马赛鼠疫暴发时穷人比富人的感染率更高，这些都不是没有原因的。有些国家和地区摆脱了利于传染性疾病滋生的环境，有些却没有。

如今持续性流行病多存在于被称为"全球南方"（Global South）的地区。流行病的阵地转移了：结核曾是欧洲致死率最高的疾病，它并没有从地球上消失，只是换了地方继续祸害人间。在有效的治疗和预防措施问世前很久，结核在西方的发病率就已经开始下降，原因是隔离等公共卫生措施的实施和生活质量的普遍改善。抗生素是现代生物医学的成就之一，它可以杀灭病菌并治愈患者，而即使在抗生素面世后，发展中国家的结核感染率仍然大幅增加。之所以会如此，是因为存在适合病菌生存的社会环境：医疗资源分配不均、居住环境拥挤、传染率高、有艾滋病等合并症，诸如此类。世界上有些国家结核的患病率在没有医学手段的干预下逐渐下降，而在另一些国家，结核在医疗干预下仍愈演愈烈。

这并不意味着药物和医学研究对控制流行病来说不重要。

3 它们的重要性毋庸置疑。抗逆转录病毒疗法不论从何种意义上说都是一项伟大的发明，它是对抗艾滋病的有力武器。然而并非所有患者都有条件得到治疗，在一些国家艾滋病的感染率正在上升。自1960年代问世以来，针对霍乱的口服补液疗法挽救了无数生命，却无法解释为何来自发展中国家的数百万人饮用的是被人类粪便污染过的水。一个明显的事实是疾病和社会状况有关，这些社会状况存在于某些国家当中，医疗措施并不能消除它。

流行病的特点是会让人感到恐惧。19世纪的霍乱引发了民众的恐慌；近代在美国等国家出现的艾滋病患者激起了人们的恐惧并遭到歧视——这种情况持续至今，如今这种疾病仍被污名化。14世纪鼠疫的暴发引发了针对犹太人的屠杀。2014年埃博拉病毒暴发期间，蔓延于美国的恐惧情绪与实际风险并不符。然而，可能导致大量死亡的流感（1918年的流行病在不到一年的时间里夺去了至少5 000万人的生命）却似乎很少造成恐慌。害怕某些特定的病与疾病的症状或染病原因有关：霍乱是一种可怕的病，它的症状很剧烈，在敏感的人看来甚至令人恶心；艾滋病和复杂的性向纠缠在一起，许多人认为艾滋病的根源是包括注射毒品在内的社会反常行为。疾病的源头也会影响人们对它的态度。疟疾是来自发展中国家的热带病。当发达国家出现散发疟疾病例时，它是以令人生畏的外来入侵者的形象出现的。

易感性——谁会染病以及为什么——至关重要。在早期的美国，殖民者认为印第安人对于天花和其他一些来自旧大陆的
4 疾病来说是一块处女地。20世纪早期，人们认为南非的黑人和其他一些人种是结核易感人群，而白人对结核有免疫力。17世

纪和18世纪，黑人被作为奴隶运送到新大陆，部分是因为非洲人相比白人不容易得疟疾。在细菌学说出现之前，人们就疾病是传染导致还是瘴气（腐烂动植物产生的臭气）所带来的争论了几百年。鼠疫常被看作对罪孽的惩罚。而对这些疾病病因的解释都发生了变化。

除天花以外，这些传染病都没有被根除。只有鼠疫——鼠疫仍然存在，1990年代印度出现过鼠疫流行，而马达加斯加常有鼠疫暴发——影响的范围和程度有所减轻。而新的疾病无疑会出现。尽管本书大部分谈论的是历史，但它并不止于历史。

规模性流行病及大流行病与现代国家兴起之间的关系是显而易见的。早在15世纪，为了应对鼠疫，意大利城邦就成立了国家资助的卫生部门。19世纪的霍乱疫情促使全国施行隔离政策——这只有中央政府才能做到。强制免疫等措施也表明了这种联系。

没有密集和流动的人口不可能暴发流行病。在人类定居下来进行农业种植和商业贸易之前，这些疾病都不曾达到流行病的规模。传染性疾病必须在不同宿主间传播才能存活，而这些宿主必须是易感的。在几个世纪里，天花对北美印第安人来说是致命疾病，这正是因为有大量没有免疫性的人群存在；这些人口的数量下降后，天花自然不再肆虐。到14世纪，贸易和旅行都得到了发展，鼠疫的传播正是利用了这些条件。结核也是在条件合适的情况下暴发的：18世纪工业化的欧洲出现了人口密集的城市和工厂。艾滋病的播散依赖于人口在全球范围内的流动。1918年的流感在几个月内蔓延到全球大部分地区，也是因为新建的交通和贸易网络以及第一次世界大战带来的人口高流动性。人类、动物和昆虫的迁徙对规模性流行病和大流行病的传播来说是决定性的。

最后，人们——目击者、小说家、诗人、传记作家、政府官员、记者、历史学家、人类学家、流行病学家、国王、王后还有总统——一直在记录流行病的历史，思考它的起因、如何控制它以及人们如何应对。我们共同积累了不计其数的素材，这些素材不止对历史学家来说具有珍贵价值。我们积累了成功和失败的经验，应该对当下研究流行病的科学家很有帮助。

鼠 疫

在疾病的历史上很难找出比"鼠疫"的含义传播更广的名词了。现在我们知道它是由鼠疫杆菌引发、由带病的跳蚤——跳蚤在动物宿主死亡后会寻找人类宿主——叮咬传播的疾病。"鼠疫"一词诞生于公元6世纪拜占庭帝国发生的已知首次大流行病期间。它通常被称为"查士丁尼鼠疫",以东罗马皇帝查士丁尼的名字命名。它来源不明——可能起源于中非内陆,随后传到埃塞俄比亚,再顺着贸易网传到了拜占庭帝国,但也可能起源于亚洲。人们无法确定。公元541年,埃及海港城市培琉喜阿姆首次出现了关于鼠疫的历史记录。在两年的时间里它横扫地中海,沿岸国家无一幸免,最后抵达东边的波斯和北边的不列颠群岛。

尽管没有准确的人口统计数据,但这次疫情中显然死亡惨重。以弗所的约翰在《教会史》(*Ecclesiastical History*)中详细记录了他的见闻,当时他正巧沿着疫情蔓延的路线旅行,从君士坦丁堡到亚历山大,又从巴勒斯坦、叙利亚和小亚细亚返回。他描绘了撂荒的田地、无人采摘的葡萄种植园、流浪的动物和日复 7

一日忙着掘墓的人们。希腊历史学家普罗柯比写道，公元542年在君士坦丁堡，鼠疫一天就夺去了一万人的生命。"人类走到了灭绝的边缘。"同时代的观察员埃瓦格里估计，鼠疫造成拜占庭首都30万人丧生。这些数字令人印象深刻——它们反映出疫情的惨烈。普罗柯比和其他熟知早前疫情的观察员都认为，查士丁尼鼠疫是前所未有的。伊斯兰化之前的阿拉伯作家察觉到疫情的特殊，他们反映鼠疫对东罗马帝国人口产生了巨大影响。早期的伊斯兰作家记录了瘟疫在短期内造成伤亡无数，人们甚至放弃将死者下葬的惨状。到7世纪中期瘟疫终于播散到英国本土时，比德在自己的《教会史》中哀叹道，鼠疫"以极大的破坏力到处肆虐……夺去了无数英国人的生命"。

在两百多年的时间里，以查士丁尼鼠疫为开端，欧洲部分地区和近东遭受了十多次鼠疫的袭击。8世纪末鼠疫消失了，可能是因为所有人或老鼠都获得了免疫力。

鼠疫的影响因地而异。从大范围内来看，农村人口凋敝对拜占庭帝国经济产生的影响——通过对钱币学、纸草学、法律文书等相关资料的详细收集整理得出的结论——表明第一次鼠疫可能促成了帝国的衰亡。与此相反，鼠疫直到公元664年才播散到英国，23年后就消失了。它在英国造成的直接影响——许多人丧生、空荡荡的修道院、荒废的村庄——令人震惊，但长期影响几乎可以忽略。诺森伯兰的修道院在660年代遭受了鼠疫的惨重袭击，两代之后又恢复了欣欣向荣的景象。鼠疫似乎无法撼动肥沃的土地、王权和巨大的财富。这些结论是从极为有限的资料中得出的，当我们试图把目光投向修道院之外普通百姓的生活时，历史记录却无处可查。

8

叙利亚深受鼠疫的影响，短期和长期都是如此。载满鼠疫病人的轮船在公元542年从埃及启航，停靠在加沙、亚实基伦、安提俄克，鼠疫从这些港口又传到大马士革，之后再传播到南方。从约翰的书中我们了解到了疫情的惨状。在那之后，公元541—749年，叙利亚几乎每七年就会暴发一次鼠疫。短期来看，鼠疫造成的死亡和大量出逃让许多地方都荒无人烟。长期来看，一再暴发的疫情给农业生产和定居人口带来了不利影响。阿拉伯人四处迁徙的生活方式使得疫情不容易蔓延，从而使得游牧民族的人口数量上升。始终脆弱的农业生产力意味着作物税收的减少和游牧经济的兴起。叙利亚鼠疫暴发次数如此之多，造成的损失如此惨重，以至于到伊斯兰早期，叙利亚成了人们口中的鼠疫之国。这一印象根深蒂固。到了中世纪，人们都知道伊斯兰叙利亚曾长期遭受鼠疫的毁灭性袭击。

关于首次鼠疫大流行我们所不知道的远远多于已知的信息。随着更先进的分析工具的出现，情况可能会有转变。通过仔细研究书面资料只能得到现有的结论。历史学家必须要利用动物学、建筑学和分子生物学等学科的知识来揭开首次鼠疫之谜。

欧洲无鼠疫之患的时代随着鼠疫的再次暴发终结于1347年，这次疫情夺去了半数——可能还不止——欧洲人的性命。第二次大流行的冲击在1353年终于过去，之后的欧洲大陆再也无法回到从前。1347年鼠疫再次暴发后，它隔一段时间就会袭击欧洲和伊斯兰国家。欧洲的最后一次鼠疫在1770年暴发于俄国。第二次鼠疫大流行不是一过性的，而是严重程度、规模和影响范围各异的多次疫情。大部分学者都认为鼠疫于14世纪中期

9

从中亚传播到欧洲后就在当地扎下根来，这一观点持续了几十年的时间。而最近关于中亚气候变迁和欧洲鼠疫流行相关性的研究表明，旧有的模型可能需要修正。鼠疫可能是一再播散到欧洲的。中亚的沙鼠在气候变暖的情况下数量激增，它们到处游走，分布广泛，成为跳蚤的完美宿主。随后这些跳蚤跳到人类和家养动物身上，当时亚洲和欧洲的港口城市比如杜布罗夫尼克贸易往来繁忙，跳蚤随之被带到了欧洲。

几个世纪后欧洲人开始接受鼠疫的存在，甚至开始预测鼠疫的到来，并想出了应对鼠疫的办法。因此，人们对1348年佛罗伦萨鼠疫和1665—1666年间伦敦鼠疫的反应就大不相同，两次鼠疫造成的影响也无法相提并论。前者对佛罗伦萨来说是前所未见的疫情，后者在1660年代虽然也是灾难性事件，但对伦敦来说，人们已经和它打过交道，对这种疾病的了解也越来越多。而在第一次大流行期间，情况并非如此。疫病的暴发突如其来，没人知道究竟发生了什么。从没有人见过这种病，它很特殊，能置人于死地。它是可怕的"黑死病"。

在七年的时间里，鼠疫在欧洲肆虐，对城市和农村造成破坏性影响。最早关于鼠疫的历史记录出现在1346年的黑海港口城市卡法，随后疫病无情地传播到欧洲各地。人们需要一个解释。为什么会有这么多人丧生？这究竟是怎样造成的？人们从几个方面对病因给出了解释：天意、瘴气、接触传染、个人易感性等等，这些病因说互相有交集。就和霍乱流行一样，这些解释（特别是瘴气和接触传染）直到19世纪末期仍然在疾病传播理论中占统治地位。在黑死病期间——借由从希腊语和拉丁语原文翻译成的阿拉伯语，中世纪晚期对伽林和希波克拉底著作的重新

10

发掘正如火如荼，而臭气会致病的学说也正兴起——瘴气和接触传染这两种学说并不像日后那样水火不容。腐烂的植物释放毒气，瘴气从地面上扩散出去，人可能因此受到感染。随后这些具有传染性的人会把疾病传给他人，特别是那些容易惹病上身的人，比如有罪之人、心怀不满之人、放荡之徒和贪吃之徒。

这些对鼠疫传播路线的自然解释可以归入大众所认为的鼠疫的根源：上帝的怒火。什鲁斯伯里的拉尔夫是巴斯和威尔斯教区主教，在感染鼠疫前，他恳求教众们祈祷。1348年夏末，他写道："邻国已经遭受了来自东方的疫病的袭击，我们担心除非我们诚心诚意、不眠不休地祈祷，同样的魔爪也将会伸向我们，夺人性命。"鼠疫来源于上天旨意这种说法也得到了其他人的支持。1348年10月，巴黎医学院的老师在当时对鼠疫病因最详尽的描述中写道："疫病的根源在于天象……行星的会合和之前的排布，与日食以及月食一起，使得人们周围的空气受到严重污染，预示着死亡和饥荒的到来。"木星和火星相会尤其会造成"大量瘴气充斥于空气中"。木星使地气蒸发，而火星则将其引燃。不过，尽管这一科学解释基于观察之上，有理论作为支撑，并且坚信药物有助于控制疫情，但人们仍认为鼠疫的根源在于上帝。"我们不能忘记瘟疫乃天意，因此我们能给出的唯一忠告就是怀着谦卑之心回归上帝。"

薄伽丘在《十日谈》中生动描述了人们对鼠疫的恐惧。《十日谈》以他在佛罗伦萨的亲身经历为基础，是描绘鼠疫之下人们生活的杰出文学作品。在鼠疫病因上，薄伽丘是一个不可知论者——鼠疫可能是"天体的影响"，也可能是"上天的惩罚，表明上帝对人类堕落生活方式的义愤"。无论原因究竟是什么，"在

11

突如其来的疫病面前，人类的智慧和才智毫无用处……医生和药物都帮不上忙"。

鼠疫造成的痛苦使得人们放弃了宗教和法律的约束：没有人活着来执行它们。薄伽丘写道，住在城郊得不到治疗、没有家人也没有邻居照料的人们"像动物一样毫无尊严地"死去。人们从未遭受过这样的灾难。"天降之祸（从某种程度上说，可能也有人祸）如此残酷，在书中提到的这一年的三月到六月带来大范围毁灭性的打击……据可靠估计，佛罗伦萨城内有10万人被夺去生命。"法国观察家写道，阿维尼翁有半数人丧生，马赛有五分之四的人死去。疫病在法国蔓延期间，"如此高的死亡率使得人们因为害怕，不敢跟任何有去世亲人的人说话，因为人们发现，家中如果有一个人去世，几乎其他所有人都会接二连三地死去"。猜疑和恐惧的情绪肆虐；人们像对待牲畜一样对待染病的家人；邻居们互相回避。在城市里，人们不顾殡葬习俗，将死去的人集中埋到大坟坑里，这至少表明了短期内社会秩序的崩塌。面对着可怕的疫病人们无能为力，许多人选择了逃离，然而穆斯林相信违抗神的旨意是亵渎神明。于是有人将疫病怪罪到其他人身上。在欧洲有多达1 000个犹太社区被暴徒们摧毁。

尽管人们普遍感到无助，威尼斯和佛罗伦萨等城市仍然成立了卫生委员会来应对疫病。为了保证空气的洁净，委员会下令要冲洗下水道和收集垃圾。当人们确信鼠疫正要蔓延到佛罗伦萨来时，政府下令禁止来自热那亚和比萨的人进入城内。疫病已成事实后，人们制定卫生条例，将"可能造成或引发空气污染的腐烂物和感染者"运走。这些措施大体上都无效。鼠疫仍然蔓延开来，夺去无数人的性命。要等到至少一百年后，稍微有些成效的预防措施才开始出现——不过到那时鼠疫的势头也早已减弱了。

面对鼠疫人们做出了种种不同反应:有人试着来解释这场灾难;有人被恐惧所裹挟;有人仓皇出逃;有人怪罪于异族。而鼠疫对于人口、经济、社会习俗、文化、宗教等的长期影响则不容易发现。短期来看,鼠疫造成了大量人口死亡——最新估计约有60%的欧洲人丧生。之后一个世纪人口仍然稀少,造成劳动力短缺、工资上涨,并伴随着通货膨胀以及更多土地被开垦用以耕种的现象。人口减少短期内改变了社会经济秩序的某些方面,英国对此有完好的记录。1349年,因为劳动力短缺,恩沙姆修道院的院长和庄主不得不重新与租户签订了对租户更有利的劳资协议。1351年,牛津伯爵约翰·德维尔庄园里的农奴被免除了许多义务。在柴郡的德雷克洛皇家庄园,根据会计官约翰·德·沃德尔的记载,"由于疫情的影响",房租减少了三分之一,"租户们威胁说不减租他们就离开(如此一来房屋将被空置),减租要一直持续到状况好转和房屋价值回升"。工资上涨了,但几乎所有生活必需品的价格也出现了上涨——劳动力短缺带来需求的上涨,同样意味着商品短缺。人们要求更低的租金和更高的工资。为了应对这种局面,1349年议会通过了《劳工条例》,1351年又通过了《劳工法令》,设定工资上限,强制人们工作,而违反者将受到惩罚。政府面临着严重的劳动力短缺,迅速采取措施来打击任何试图从中获利之人。

要通过法律来阻止人们寻求高工资和低租金意味着,在黑死病结束以及14世纪随后的几十年内,人们的心态发生了一些可察的变化。精英阶层对农民行为(多被污蔑)的看法证实了

13

7

这一点。农民拿着新到手的盈余添置和身份不符的衣服;他们还开始打猎——这在以前可是富人独享的活动。

诗人约翰·高尔哀叹着旧日时光一去不回:"过去农民不常吃小麦面包;他们吃的是豆子和其他谷物粉做的面包,喝的只有水而已。有奶酪和牛奶就算是大餐了,他们难得吃到比这更好的美食。他们穿的就是普通的灰布衣裳。人们安居乐业,尊卑有序。"可现在"美好的旧时光全给毁了"。这是因为"仆人和主人全给颠倒过来了……农民学主人的样子,穿主人式样的衣服"。为了规范"与财产和地位不符的过度着装"而出台的节俭法令,也反映出农民生活方式的显著改变。黑死病过去后的几十年里,这种对人们安分守己的旧时光的哀叹很常见。尽管法律明文禁止索要和开出高工资,这种做法仍然屡见不鲜:面对着长期的劳动力短缺以及1360—1362年间和1369年疫病的雪上加霜,人们别无选择。

意大利的工人也要求提高工资。佛罗伦萨的编年史作家马泰奥·维拉尼写道:"女仆和毫无服务经验的妇人以及马房伙计都要至少12弗罗林一年,最狂妄的甚至开价要18 ~ 24弗罗林一年,护士和工匠学徒的工钱也涨到以前的三倍,种地的农民个个都要配耕牛和种子,都想种最肥的地,不要差些的地。"从政府的应对措施中我们可以看出,这不止是少数心怀不满的劳工提出的要求,这些措施包括设立工资上限、强制人们签订工作合同而不得谈条件。

尽管很难准确知道人们生活的改善情况——相关的数据哪怕有也很难找——但讽刺的是,黑死病过去后的几十年里,不论男女,的确比瘟疫前的人们生活要好些。

欧洲人口减少带来的只是短期冲击。之后一百年内,生产力和人口数量又有所恢复甚至蓬勃增长。要近两百年后地中海西部的人口才能重新恢复到疫情前的水平,而直到1600年英国的人口才恢复。不过,人口数量减少没有造成长期负面影响。有一种解释是疫前的人口数量可能已经达到了马尔萨斯人口理论所说的临界点,资源已经达到了最大负载。按照这种观点,虽然短期看来鼠疫是悲惨的,但长期看来可能对社会是有益处的。黑死病后的一个世纪里,欧洲各地实际工资的增加有史可查,这可以用人工费用上涨来解释。将如此辽阔地域上的经济和人口变迁归结为单个事件的影响,即使这个事件破坏巨大,也是不可能的,甚至概括总结都很困难。许多改变可能已经在悄然发生:到处都出现了人口减少;许多地方的劳工关系和土地所有制在疫情之前就有所变化——12世纪和13世纪毫无疫情影响,而那时农奴制在佛兰德斯和荷兰就已经消亡。不过另一方面,鼠疫可能将科技发展的步伐往前推了一百多年。风车和水车等动力设施发展迅猛,枪械的使用也是如此。是鼠疫暴发导致人口减少,人们才开始使用这些工具的吗?有可能。就算鼠疫不是社会变迁的唯一因素,它肯定加速了变化的到来,这似乎是不可否认的。

如此大规模的疫情在文学、艺术和宗教上都留下了印记。鼠疫之后,有些地方的人们表现出极度的虔诚,而另一些地方爆发了对宗教约束的反抗。中欧的苦修者——一群笃信宗教的信徒,他们表达虔诚的独特方式包括当众鞭笞自己——开始承担牧师的传统职责,宣扬上帝即将来到人间,会把富人的财富分给穷人,让世上再没有压迫。艺术作品对死亡这一主题的迷恋反映出人们意识到了死亡的不可预知性。鼠疫后大学得到了发展——牧师人手不足、疫后人们沉溺于学习都促进了大学的建立。在英国，人们不再修建规模宏大的教堂，改为修建朴实的小教堂。

黑死病暴发几十年和几百年后，医生有了经验，死亡率有所下降，政府也在疫病的控制中发挥了更积极的作用。在许多地方，疫病规律性地暴发，使得人们慢慢适应了疫病的存在。1500—1665年伦敦暴发了17次鼠疫。1500—1720年近三百年的时间里，法国每年都暴发鼠疫。埃及每8～9年就会经历一次鼠疫；从黑死病暴发到1517年被奥斯曼帝国占领，叙利亚-巴勒斯坦暴发了18次大规模的鼠疫。鼠疫成了常态，而且之后再也没有出现过像黑死病那样席卷整个欧洲大陆的惨烈疫情，这意味着人们的恐慌情绪减少了许多，也不再将灾难怪罪于别人。和黑死病期间针对犹太人的袭击事件层出不穷相反，之后的一个世纪里只在波兰发生过一起袭击。黑死病的恐怖没有重演；鼠疫仍然很可怕，但成了平常之事。医生和市政当局有了更多信心来应对疫病。尽管人们无法预知疫病何时何地会暴发——就像一位历史学家所说，鼠疫"有种令人费解的随机性"——但它仍然表现出某种大致规律：它首先袭击港口，接着是内陆城市，然后从城市蔓延到农村。疫病出现在城市的特定街区，挨家挨户地传播，似乎毫无规律可循。疫情之下能看出人们的行为模式，许多人选择逃离疫区。人们都想保全自己，这也意味着有些时候会弃他人于不顾。大体说来，政府仍保持完好，鼠疫也没有造成社会秩序的崩塌。早期现代欧洲各地政府应对疫病的措施——成立政府资助的卫生委员会、医院、鼠疫隔离医院以及采取隔离机制——巩固了国家的统治。

随着医生不再相信鼠疫是上帝的怒火或是行星的排列所致，

大流行病

控制疫病的手段也开始变化。医生试着找出更切实际的病因并且治愈疾病。14世纪末，医生开始认为鼠疫促进了医学的进步，15世纪这种观点进一步得到发展。治疗鼠疫过程中采用的各种疗法让医生积累了丰富的临床经验，这在中世纪晚期出现的一类专门讨论鼠疫病因的鼠疫论著作中有翔实的记载。有几次疫情相对轻微，人们可以在大暴发时所不允许的不那么紧迫和危急的情况下从容地开展研究。医生的信心得到提升，许多人宣称自己的医术超过了希波克拉底和伽林等古代医家，声称这些前辈没有和鼠疫打过交道，而他们自己攻克了鼠疫。

黑死病后再没有发生过如此大规模的死亡。严重的疫情仍有发生——1656—1657年间热那亚市有60%的人死去，还有至少六次疫情夺去了马赛、帕多瓦和米兰等地30%的人的性命。大多数情况下死亡率都有所下降。死亡率的显著下降和人们对医疗技术信心的提升是相符的。这些信心部分当然来自对疾病有了新的了解，比如知道隔离病人的必要性。但也有可能随着人群慢慢产生了免疫，疫情的严重程度逐渐减轻。

传染这一观念有着悠久的历史。它的发展历程充满曲折，从伽林提出传染源理论一直延续到文艺复兴时期；其间在阿拉伯世界瘟疫的病因学说上，传染让位于瘴气和上帝降罪理论；直到16世纪在欧洲，传染理论才重新获得了发展。早在14世纪晚期就出现了鼠疫可能有传染性这一论断。黑死病在地中海造成惨重破坏期间，阿拉伯作家伊本·哈提卜旗帜鲜明地表达了对传染理论的支持。他的观点和穆斯林世界普遍接受的上帝降罪理论相悖。他写道："若要问我为何接受神意早已否定的传染一说，我将这样作答：经验、推断、常识、观察以及无数报告都证实了传染的存在,上述种种皆可作为证据。"

现代欧洲早期出现的传染理论常常和瘴气学说共存,而上帝的影响仍然无处不在。比如英国牧师理查德·利克就不接受任何除神意之外的病因理论。他吟诵道:"不是空气污染、瘟热,更非女巫的恶毒行径、霉运或其他任何臆想的原因,而是我们自身的罪孽才招致这些灾祸。"鼠疫是上帝降罪于人间的。1630年秋,鼠疫袭击了托斯卡纳内陆地区一个名叫蒙特卢坡的小村。政府官员和宗教领袖就鼠疫的原因和应当采取的措施争论不休。和其他大多数居民一样,宗教领袖主张举行游行来平息上帝的怒火。政府部门的卫生官员认为鼠疫有传染性,试图阻止公众集会,并将病人和他们的家属隔离起来。暴乱随之爆发。在西班牙和意大利,弗朗西斯科·瓦莱斯、维托雷·丁卡雷拉和吉罗拉莫·弗拉卡斯托罗等作家都指出鼠疫这类疾病有传染性。正如瓦莱斯评论伽林的《流行病学》时所说,"如果没有传染物质从患者传播到被感染者,那鼠疫这类传染病是无法产生的。此乃众所周知,盖因所有活动都必须通过接触才能发生……必然有传染源从病人传给被感染者,这种传染源即某种污秽之物"。不过早期传染理论和现代传染理论有着天壤之别。1636年,英国评论家斯蒂芬·布拉德维尔在写作中很自然地将传染和瘴气混为一谈,因为在研究鼠疫(或其他疾病)病因论的这个阶段,两者并不是水火不容的:正如他所写的,"人们可以将自身疾病通过接触传给他人,不管这种接触是通过肉身、精神抑或是呼吸来达成的"。这种传染媒介是"有毒酊剂,它质地轻盈,含有酒精,能和空气混合在一起,穿透毛孔"。

政府开始对人们和货物采取隔离措施,颁布旅行禁令,禁止宗教游行等公众集会,将患者和疑似病人纳入更有力的政府控制之下,这些举措表明传染理论得到了(部分)认可。在率先施行这些措施的意大利北部,卫生委员会在疫情期间施行了和公共卫生相关的法律。不过这些措施收效甚微,鼠疫仍然横行。 19

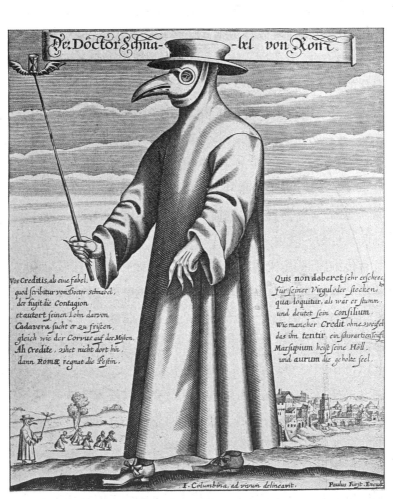

图1 这幅1656年的版画刻画了鼠疫医生的标志性形象,他头戴装有草药的鸟嘴保护面罩来阻挡瘟疫的传播

然而这些举措可能反映出并强化了疾病和贫穷的关联。在意大利、法国和英国，人们发现穷人比富人更容易遭受鼠疫的袭击。1720年马赛的最后一次大疫病暴发期间，一位医生就富裕街区这样写道："街道开阔，房屋宽敞，所住的都是富人，因为有办法尽量逃离疫病的魔爪，他们往往也是最不容易感染的人。"当时许多人相信鼠疫会传染并且穷人才会得病，富人越来越担心疫病会跨阶层传染。鼠疫变成了一个社会问题，它成了贫富分化的标志。对鼠疫的恐惧和对穷人的恐惧如影相随。

　　随着欧洲国家开始对货物实行强制检疫隔离，鼠疫的传染性对经济也产生了影响。海上检疫的历史可以追溯到14世纪末期，杜布罗夫尼克是最早实行检疫的港口城市。尽管这项措施引发了争议，效果也常常不明显，但仍渐渐成为常规。不光货物需要隔离，旅客也可能会而且的确常常被隔离起来。贸易、旅行和鼠疫的关联由来已久。因为许多人认为鼠疫发源于东方并且有传染性，扣留来自东方的货物和旅客的做法自然深得人心。穆斯林国家的情况却并非如此，人们对传染理论的接受程度更低，而奥斯曼帝国也不具备施行隔离的行政能力。印度和中国这些常常被认为是鼠疫发源地的国家也没有施行检疫措施。因此欧洲国家特别是地中海沿岸国家自己在边境设立了检疫机构。鼠疫发源于东方，可这些国家没有采取任何措施来阻止疾病的传播，这种观念加剧了东西方的分歧——19世纪霍乱暴发期间分歧变得更加不可调和。

　　并不是所有国家都严格地执行检疫隔离措施，这样做的是那些更靠近疫源地的国家。同样重要的是国家的管理实力和保护人民免受疫病侵袭能力这两者的联系越来越紧密。这种关联在意大利独立城邦表现得最明显，1575—1578年鼠疫肆虐于 全意大利境内时更是发挥了巨大作用。意大利通过改良卫生状况、限制人口和货物（特别是境外人口和货物）的流动来阻止疫病播散，这些举措加深了人们对疫源的了解，开创性地成立许多卫生部门也使得意大利与众不同。不过，这些做法渐渐在欧洲其他国家也流行起来——1578年英国的首个鼠疫法令就明显受到了意大利的影响——特别是检疫和隔离变得越来越普遍。

尽管国家为了控制疫情采取了种种措施，但因为执法不严、边境管理松懈、商人为了生存违反规定等原因，效果没有完全显现。另外，意大利这些城邦都很小，长期以来人们拥有强烈的公民自豪感和自我保护意识。而在国家更为庞大、人口组成复杂的法国，建立检疫制度难度很大。甚至当人们采取了海上检疫措施，比如1664年鼠疫从低地国家传播到伦敦期间所做的那样，它也并不总是收效，在这一年和之后两年里，伦敦遭受了一个世纪多以来最惨重的鼠疫袭击。理论上说，病人居家隔离是一个好办法，实际上却没有任何帮助：病人们不遵守居家的命令，而这样的人数不胜数。18世纪，作为一种公共卫生措施，隔离及其对商业的影响遭到了相当的质疑，它越来越像是愚昧时代残留的糟粕。

假如说第二波鼠疫暴发的时间可以精确到1347年和黑死病的到来，疫病消失的时间却无法精确到哪一年。它逐渐式微，从一个个国家消失不见，再也无法卷土重来。英国最后一次鼠疫暴发于1665—1666年间，夺去了八万伦敦居民的性命。半个世纪后，在马赛出现了西欧最后一次鼠疫。50年后莫斯科出现了欧洲最后一波疫情。整个18世纪埃及不断遭受鼠疫的袭击，

1791年大流行期间，开罗30万人中有20%丧生。奥斯曼帝国直到19世纪仍在遭受瘟疫袭击。在三百多年的时间里，鼠疫对宗教信仰、疾病的传播理论、人口和经济都产生了影响；它促进了首个国家资助的公共卫生措施的问世。接着鼠疫就消失了。从早期现代世界范围来看，鼠疫似乎是渐渐消失的——毕竟伦敦和莫斯科的最后一次疫病隔了一百多年。不过从局部或者国家范围来看，疫病似乎是突然消失的。自1340年代以来，英国不断受到鼠疫侵袭。1665—1666年最后一次大暴发后，鼠疫就一去不返。法国的情况也是如此：在几个世纪里，几乎每年都会暴发鼠疫，而1720年马赛的疫病暴发后就再也不见鼠疫的踪影。这是怎么回事呢？可能是老鼠产生了免疫力，阻断了鼠疫的传播，也可能是占主导地位的老鼠种类变了。可能是造成鼠疫再三播散的中亚气候波动稳定下来。另外，尽管许多情况下隔离措施效果并不明显，但长远来看，它的作用开始显现，从而逐渐阻止了疫病的传播。从1666年起，英国开始严格实行隔离政策，鼠疫再也没有卷土重来。然而鼠疫持续时间长，影响的地区众多而且千差万别，最后消失的时间也各异，因此很难确定疾病消亡的唯一原因。

1890年代鼠疫再次暴发时，历史的记忆仍然鲜活。19世纪霍乱的流行唤起了曾经历过鼠疫的国家的记忆，让它们回想起阻击疫病的情景；霍乱期间所采取的措施大都是在第二次鼠疫流行期间发展起来的。它的影响极为深远。同样，霍乱也影响了之后第三次鼠疫暴发时人们的应对方式。

1890年第三次鼠疫大流行在华南暴发。疫病沿着珠江播散到广东，随后抵达南方最大的贸易城市——广州。之后又传

23

播到邻近的香港以及更远的地区。1890年代疫病扩散到了许多国家和地区，主要集中在海港城市。开普敦、悉尼、火奴鲁鲁和旧金山都暴发了鼠疫。里约热内卢和布宜诺斯艾利斯也未能幸免。在葡萄牙的波尔图，海上检疫措施让经济活动陷入了停滞。虽然这些城市的死亡率并不高，人们却陷入了极度恐慌当中——八万人逃离香港；在开普敦和悉尼，隔离成为对非洲黑人和华人施行种族政策的手段；旧金山和火奴鲁鲁对华人采取了严厉的措施。疫病肆虐于印度北部和西部大部分地区，造成近1 200万人死亡。1914年塞内加尔遭到了鼠疫第三次袭击，之后30年里疫病动摇了法国在这片殖民地上的统治地位。1910年中国东北境内暴发了一种致命的肺鼠疫。

第三次鼠疫大流行并非说明黑死病卷土重来。除不容忽视的印度外，这次疫病的病死率大大降低——疾病的凶险程度可能有所减轻，公共卫生措施也更加有力。疫情监控、海上检疫、病人隔离——政府采取上述所有以及其他措施来控制疫病，有时近乎残暴和铁腕。在埃及的亚历山大市，卫生官员们摒弃了强迫人们遵守严格的公共卫生措施的做法，让民间领袖参与进来，赢得了人们的信任和主动合作。如此一来避免了大面积的恐慌，市内的疫病在几个月内就得到了控制。

不断提速的蒸汽船和大量增加的铁路使得全球贸易网快速发展，人口的迁移也越来越频繁，导致在短时间内疫病就扩散到 24 了世界各地。商业、人口迁移和传染性疾病的关联——以及设法实现国际合作来对抗疫病的必要性——在19世纪的霍乱大流行中表现得非常明显。这种关联性在鼠疫卷土重来和1918年大流感席卷全球期间变得更为明显。

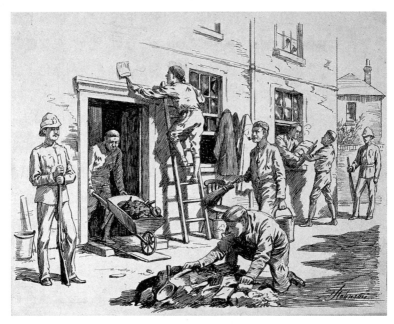

图2　1891年第三次鼠疫大流行期间，囚犯们在给开普敦市消毒

　　在科学家得到重大的实验室发现时，鼠疫再次暴发。1894
年疫病暴发早期，瑞士裔法国科学家亚历山大·耶尔森和日本
研究员北里柴三郎分别发现了鼠疫杆菌，两人前后相差十天。
随后，随着疫病在全球播散，鼠疫由老鼠身上的跳蚤所传播这一
25　理论也流传开来。这一理论最初由法国科学家保罗-路易·西
蒙于1898年在孟买工作期间提出。哪些人会感染鼠疫、感染方
式如何、鼠疫又是怎样传播，这些讨论是几个世纪以来和鼠疫有
关著作的主题，现在终于尘埃落定。

　　鼠疫杆菌的发现以一种有些突然的方式从本质上改变了人
们对鼠疫的认知。1890年鼠疫暴发，1894年科学家在显微镜下
发现了鼠疫杆菌，因此鼠疫现在成了一种可知的明确的疾病，尽

管仍有些令人触摸不着；而自6世纪以来造成生灵涂炭的鼠疫，过去在人们眼中一直是虚无缥缈、神秘莫测的。鼠疫杆菌的发现改变了一切，人们在回顾时可以根据患者的症状确认曾经的疫病正是鼠疫杆菌所致。耶尔森和北里柴三郎都声称发现了中世纪鼠疫的病因。以实验研究为基础的现代鼠疫理论将被应用到对古老疾病的解释上。不久之后鼠疫杆菌正式被命名为鼠疫耶尔森氏菌（*Yersinia pestis*）。

对鼠疫的新认知带来了回顾性诊断这一问题。我们如何确认在542年袭击君士坦丁堡、1349年造访阿维尼翁以及1665年席卷伦敦的，正是现知的由鼠疫耶尔森氏菌所引起的鼠疫呢？有些历史学家和生物学家对此予以否认，他们着重指出了疾病严重程度的可能差异；他们声称老鼠的迁徙不够快，不可能造成疫病如此快速地蔓延。有些病人没有鼠疫样症状，而且没有老鼠大规模死亡的证据。这些学者的观点建立在现代鼠疫和中世纪鼠疫两者的不同之上。他们认为两者区别明显，不可能是同一种疾病。

而认为两者是同一疾病的观点是以两者的相同点为基础的：两者症状一样，特别是都有标志性的名为淋巴结炎的腋窝、腹股沟和颈部肿大。几乎可以确定，在许多出现过鼠疫的地区，老鼠和跳蚤都很猖獗。和现代鼠疫一样，历史上的鼠疫——就我们所知——先是通过海运传播的，表明船上有老鼠存在。鼠疫理论的支持者们还指出，病菌会演化，历史上鼠疫的症状在某些方面和第三次鼠疫大流行有区别也就不奇怪了。那历史上的疫病究竟是什么？迄今为止，大多数历史学家、遗传学家和分子生物学家都认为所有的疫病都是鼠疫耶尔森氏菌所致。原因之

26

一是从古代、中世纪晚期和现代早期的坟墓中收集到的DNA样本证实了这一点。

自从热那亚人和东方开展贸易从而引起1340年代鼠疫的首次暴发，鼠疫和贸易的关系就为人所熟知。1850年代到19世纪末，新兴的国际社会定期召开一系列国际卫生大会来讨论如何控制传染性疾病的传播。第三次鼠疫大流行暴发时，科学国际主义正达到高潮，而1897年在威尼斯召开的国际卫生大会就证明了这一点，会上有关鼠疫的最新科学发现迎合了人们对放松贸易管制的长久期盼。科学或能服务于贸易。

在威尼斯会议上，国际社会达成了前所未有的共识。伦敦流行病学会会长称在这次会议中，"国际社会在形成关于传染病防控措施的**开明**和**科学**的观念方面取得了长足进展"。随着疫情监控和上报等更有效措施的应用，隔离措施慢慢不再流行。一旦疫病的暴发地得到确认，政府就能够在当地采取限制人口流动或海港检疫等更有针对性的举措，而不是在恐惧和无知的驱使下限制所有贸易。并非所有国家都遵守了会议公约——葡萄牙和西班牙采用的是在港口实行无效的军事封锁等传统更僵化的措施——但在埃及等遵守共识的国家，贸易禁令很快得以解除。六年后在巴黎举行的卫生大会上，该共识仍有效力。那时人们开始关注会携带鼠疫病菌的老鼠，关注焦点也转向阻止鼠疫从始发港向外传播。这取决于当地政府的能力和对两件事的重视程度，这两件事是公认的控制鼠疫的必要措施：卫生改革和强有力的疾病监控及上报系统。在世界范围内，这两项政策的实施并不均衡。

科学和贸易的关系在印度表现得很明显，这个国家无疑是

27

第三次鼠疫期间遭受打击最惨重的。1896年鼠疫在孟买暴发，一开始疫病就对英属殖民地的疫情防控能力提出了极大的挑战，对医学新建立的信心提出了质疑。起初，政府以前所未有的力度介入和干预印度人民的生活，并以1897年《传染病法案》的颁布告终。为了响应国际社会的呼声，阻止疫病蔓延到欧洲，殖民地官员被赋予了极大的权力，负责施行登船检查、社区隔离、颁布旅行和宗教集会禁令以及实施卫生措施。法案允许当局采取任何可能有效的举措。殖民地官员给予了医生和卫生专家前所未有的影响力，让他们参与政策制定，医学技术也随之树立了权威。

这些政策——熏蒸和焚烧房屋；强制将病人送往不顾种姓习俗、人人畏惧的医院；禁止举办葬礼；对死者进行尸检；严格隔离病人等等——引发了19世纪印度历史上对西方医学最大规模的抵制。

浦那的一份英文报纸《马拉地人》(*Mahratta*) 写道，英国人从未如此"有组织地大规模地介入印度人的家庭、社交和宗教生活"。家庭隔离特别是将妇女带往隔离营是人们最憎恨的做法之一，也引发了最暴力的反抗。在浦那，英国士兵当街检查妇女、频繁搜查房屋的做法也引发众怒，导致防疫指挥官 W.C. 兰德在1897年6月被暗杀。此后一年，政府采取了更多措施，反抗也达到了顶峰：印度北部各地都爆发了反对搜查房屋、隔离政策和强制入院的骚乱。

殖民政府不得不做出让步——阻击疫病和镇压抗议影响了殖民地的经济；使用武力只能适得其反。或许和印度人民合作比镇压的效果会更好。卫生指挥官认识到，"经验告诉我们，可取的医疗措施实际上可能不可行,并且会带来危险的政治后果"。

在政府做出转变后,即使在曾爆发最激烈抗议的浦那,人们也开始表现出和殖民地官员合作的态度。1900年印度鼠疫委员会发布了一份报告,报告中说政府态度从强迫转变为合作卓有成效。人们的抵抗表明了对西方医学缺乏信心,新时代的合作也突显出人们意识到那些英国官员虽然表面上吵吵嚷嚷,实际上心中也没有答案。此后殖民地官员再也不可能以这种方式将观点强加给印度人民。认为这标志着印度迎来了合作和平等时代的曙光的观点,将会被印度国内事态的发展所推翻。重点在于英国殖民政府对鼠疫的最初应对表明,这是一个只会把观点强加给人民的政权。一旦武力的使用适得其反,英国政府不得不接受失败命运,殖民政府和西方医学并不像他们所标榜的那样强大这一点也就昭然若揭。

到第一次世界大战爆发时,各国的鼠疫疫情要么得到了控制,要么已经开始消退。但鼠疫并没有消失。尽管现在可以用抗生素来治疗,但治疗必须争分夺秒,又因为鼠疫有传染性,它可以在很短的时间内传播开来。鼠疫在非洲和亚洲的一些地区断断续续时有出现,持续几十年的时间;1990年代印度和21世纪早期马达加斯加鼠疫的暴发提醒人们,这种古老而令人闻之色变的疾病仍未远去。不过它再也没有达到全球流行的程度。

天 花

在1980年世界卫生组织宣布消灭天花前，它作为一种规模性流行病和大流行病，已经肆虐了近千年的时间，甚至可能更久。来自埃及木乃伊身上的证据有趣但不具有确定性；修昔底德所描述的发端于公元前430年令人难忘的雅典鼠疫可能是天花。数亿人因此病而丧生。最早最详尽的关于天花的描述来自公元4世纪的中国药学家葛洪，他在《肘后备急方》中写道，"比岁有病时行，仍发疮头面及身，须臾周匝，状如火疮，皆戴白浆，随决随生"。生活在公元10世纪巴格达的波斯医生拉齐著有《天花与麻疹》一书，其中关于天花的描述流传最广，对天花救治的影响延续到17世纪。中国、印度和非洲许多地区发现的证据都表明，天花和人类共存了几个世纪。印度北部大部分地区，特别在18世纪和19世纪，人们将天花视为神灵而非疾病，天花女神名为湿陀罗。1830年代或许更早，切诺基人发明了名叫 *itohvnv* 的舞蹈，来平息以天花现身人世的邪灵（名为 Kosvkvsini）的怒火。西非的约鲁巴人和其他部落信奉天花之

31

神。1770年代天花大规模暴发后，南非科萨人不再举行葬礼仪式；感染者在灌木丛中独自死去，无人照料。死亡不再是生命自然的一部分，而是面目狰狞、令人胆寒的存在。日本的阿伊努人认为天花是沟通天地之神，它把人变成鬼，在人间散播疾病。天花这样一种造成惨重伤亡的疾病会深刻地影响人们的心理也在意料之中。

非洲的奴隶贸易和定居者的殖民政策将天花带到了美洲，它和其他一些疾病使得多达90%的土著丧生。16世纪早期到19世纪中期，因为大量易感人群的存在，天花造成了一连串致死性的规模性流行，并演变成了延续几世纪的全球大流行。

确定美洲土著感染的疾病很有难度。许多疾病都很相似，都有发烧、身体不适或咳嗽等症状。目击者的描述可能太模糊。不过，天花的独特症状，特别是葛洪首先描述的脓疱，使得识别天花比仅依靠殖民时代的简单描述来区分其他一些疾病（比如肺炎和肺结核）要容易得多。天花的症状对大部分当代观察家来说都清晰无误——到16世纪和17世纪天花已经是欧洲大多数地区孩子们常得的病——因此他们不再用疫病或瘟疫而是直接用天花来称呼这些流行疾病。墨西哥人没有相应的词汇来描述他们从未见过的疾病，但1520年《佛罗伦萨法典》中的记录表明，正是天花使得阿兹特克首都特诺其蒂特兰的人们大量死去，城市随后才被西班牙人占领。

人群中暴发了一种可怕的疾病并且蔓延开来。疫病肆虐，夺去了无数人的生命。感染的人们全身布满脓疱：头上、脸上和胸膛上到处都是。境况凄惨无比。人们动弹不

32

得，连转头或是动一动都无法做到。脓疮带来了巨大的痛苦，病人不能趴，不能躺，也不能翻身。当他们试着挪动身体的时候，会因为疼痛而大叫。许多人因此丧生，还有许多人活活饿死。而他们之所以饿死是因为已经无人再来照顾他们。许多人被毁容；他们变成了麻子，脸上坑坑洼洼，会伴随一生。还有人瞎了眼，双目失明。病情最厉害的阶段会持续60天，整整60天的恐怖。

由此看来，天花不容易和别的病混淆（尽管有时候区分天花和麻疹会很困难）。

像天花这种疾病，直到17世纪末在欧洲都并不特别致命，为何在美洲却夺去众多性命呢？新英格兰早期的殖民者认为是上帝为了惩罚他们异教徒的生活方式并且清理人口，才将疾病和死亡带给印第安人的。清教徒编年史作家威廉·布拉德福德在回顾1633年的天花流行时写道，"给印第安人带来疾病合乎上帝的心意"。这样一来，"上帝赋予我们对这片土地的所有权"。在弗吉尼亚州的罗阿诺克，托马斯·哈利奥特写道，阿尔冈昆人认为"疫病是上帝的旨意，借人之手来实施，在神的帮助下我们可以不费片甲杀光一切敌人"。休伦人则怪罪于法国人。据1630年代末天花大暴发后一名耶稣会传教士所写，休伦人觉得法国人是"地球上最厉害的巫师"，这些人所到之处，休伦人纷纷丧命，而传教士则安然无恙。

历史学家常常把人口大规模死亡归因为所谓的处女地流行病。这种观点很简单：欧洲的儿童常见病对那些从未接触过的人来说就是夺命杀手。处女地的说法也延续了基因和种族的共同作用造就更强壮或更孱弱的民族这一观念。事实并非如此。在被某种疾病感染之前，所有的人群都毫无抵抗力。1713年的处女地流行病中，南非的科伊桑人饱受天花之苦；1707—1709年间，一次天花流行夺去了冰岛这片"处女地"上三分之一冰岛人的性命。这一概念带给我们的启示是，天花等疾病在许多成员都缺乏免疫力的人群中会造成灾难性后果，起初是新大陆的原住民，后来是18世纪早期的科伊桑人，再后来是间隔几十年的数次流行侵袭下的大部分冰岛居民。处女地这一说法可以极好地解释美洲印第安人对天花等疾病的易感性，但它只能用来解释对从未遭遇过的疾病的早期易感性。

天花的毁灭性影响还可以用其他因素解释。有可能美洲印第安人在与世隔绝千年之后形成的基因同质性使得他们更易感；也有可能新大陆的天花来源于非洲而非欧洲，因此毒性更厉害。天花被再三地带到新大陆，而每次流行之间都有着时间间隔，这意味新的流行在许多地方袭来时，上一次流行的幸存者业已死去。许多人群的人口数量较少，天花不足以形成流行以使人群获得免疫力（这一现象也可以解释20世纪早期天花在肯尼亚的游牧民族中造成的惨重伤亡）。一个社群中只要有足够的缺乏免疫力的人口，天花就会持续为害。未感染过的母亲没有抗体可以遗传给后代，而母亲一旦患病也无法照顾染病的孩子。许多印第安人的村庄都人口稠密；更甚者一大群人常常住在一个屋檐下——为天花快速传播创造了完美条件。由于没有传染的概念，健康人会去看望病人。人们因为恐慌纷纷逃离，天花就这样播散开来。

大量人口死亡带来的混乱导致许多人因饥饿和脱水而死。

34

1630年代,威廉·布拉德福德在描述天花幸存者的生存境况时写道:"这些人境遇悲惨,疾病感染太过普遍以致最后他们无力互相扶持,连生火或是弄点水喝或是掩埋死者都做不到。"天花流行是带来深重灾难的殖民地运动的产物。1696—1700年的东南部天花大流行是因为当地奴隶贸易带来的混乱和人口持续流动才成为可能的。在几十年的时间里,奴隶贸易通过劫掠和迁徙扰乱了当地人民的生活。

天花重塑了北美印第安部落的分布情况。自1630年代以来的一个多世纪里,欧洲人与土著之间的河狸皮、枪支和酒精贸易促进了天花的播散,给五大湖区和平原/牧场交界地带带来了改变。1630年代遭受天花的毁灭性打击后,易洛魁人向宿敌休伦人发起了更多的"哀悼之战"——俘获敌人来代替本族的死者。天花给易洛魁人造成了巨大的破坏,却几乎给休伦人带来灭顶之灾。另外,由于易洛魁人强大的军事实力,他们成了这一区域的霸主。这次疫情迫使索克人和福克斯人为寻找藏身之处逃往更西方的部族中间,促进了新民族的产生。天花不断卷土重来,一次次重塑了各民族的版图。死亡率的差异使得有些部族渐渐式微,有些变得强大。1670年代,说阿尼士纳比语的蒙索尼人成为很有势力的皮毛贸易中间商,而在1730年代的天花疫情中他们却几乎被灭族;幸存者流落到其他部族中,到18世纪末期蒙索尼人已经不再是独立的民族。他们像北奥吉布瓦人一样消失了。

1780年代早期,墨西哥城暴发了疫病并一路向北蔓延,抵达哈德逊湾和太平洋西北部。最初的慌乱平息后,南部平原上的科曼奇人躲开了疫病的袭击:他们没有旅行前往疫病多发的商业中心,而是待在家里等着生意上门。躲开天花袭击以及另外一些原因使得科曼奇人成为18世纪到19世纪中期最强大、人口最多的美洲印第安部族。北部平原上，密苏里河沿岸的村庄几乎被疫病损毁殆尽。阿里卡拉部落人口减少了80%。1795年，法国商人让-巴蒂斯特·特吕托写道："历史上阿里卡拉是大部族；共有32个人口稠密的村庄，不同时期数次天花袭击过后，村子里人烟稀少，几乎全部被毁。每村只有几个家庭逃过一劫。"

平原上骑马的民族，特别是西苏族，因为地理的庇佑躲过了最严重的疫病，在竞争中占了上风。到1800年，整个大平原地区都被马背上的游猎民族所占领。密苏里河沿岸的村庄被大量损毁。1804年11月，威廉·克拉克和梅利韦瑟·路易斯造访平原地区时写道："许多年前，他们住在密苏里沿岸的数个村庄里，天花夺去了大多数人的性命，只留存下一个大村子和一些小村子。疫情之前其他民族都很忌惮他们，而在他们衰落后，苏族和其他部落发动了战争，杀人无数，他们只得沿密苏里河而上。"

直到19世纪印第安人仍饱受天花之苦。1837—1838年的疫病几乎使得曼丹人、希多特萨人和阿里卡拉人被灭绝；同一次疫病向西蔓延，摧毁了黑脚、大肚和阿西尼博因部族。而日益强大的拉科塔人、夏安人和阿拉帕霍人组成的联盟占领了这些无人之境。当19世纪中期不断增加的美国人向西部腹地挺进时，他们所发现的由科曼奇人、拉科塔人、阿拉帕霍人和夏安人统治的印第安世界其实是在天花影响下形成的。

在早期现代欧洲，天花是常见病，它在许多地方都很流行，在另一些地方则进一步播散成为大规模流行病。17世纪中期以前，天花并不是厉害的致死性疾病。它是低风险的流行病，在教科书或者编年史作家和旅行家的记录中，很少会作为危险疾病

36

出现。大范围的疫情没有出现过。在16世纪晚期的伦敦，因天花而死的情况很罕见，而且死亡的都是孩子。然而随后天花发生了变异。18世纪天花成为欧洲致死率最高的疾病，在人们心中造成的恐慌和致死率都超过了鼠疫。1649年开始暴发，并且在17世纪后半叶每隔一段时间就卷土重来，天花疫情导致的死亡人数在伦敦年死亡人数中占比超过8%。到18世纪中期这个数字翻了一番：1762年天花夺去了3 500人的生命，占伦敦死亡人数的17%。到18世纪末天花使得8%～20%的人口死亡。

随着接种和疫苗的出现，情况出现了转机。接种是在伤口上接入少量病毒，以引发身体低水平的免疫反应。如果一切顺利，病人会有轻微的天花症状并且获得终身免疫，就和得过病的幸存者一样。早在18世纪中期接种于欧洲流行起来以前，非洲、印度和中国一些地区的人们就采用了这种方法。18世纪早期，关于接种疗效的新闻慢慢传到了英国人和美国人耳中——波士顿的科顿·马瑟牧师告诉人们，一名来自西非的奴隶说这种做法很普遍；中国人接种天花的消息在1700年传到了英国；17世纪波兰和丹麦的农民开始接种的消息也流传开来。1718年，英国驻土耳其大使夫人玛丽·沃特利·蒙塔古在接种已经被人们熟知的君士坦丁堡给女儿接种了天花，之后接种开始流行起来；1721年她的儿子成为英国首个接种天花的人。英国皇室也很快开始接受接种，天花接种成为医院的普遍做法。

不过也出现了反对的声音，人们担心接种会带来危险，宗教人士担心接种会改变命运。这些反对意见得到了有力反击：接种使得更多人产生免疫，挽救了生命。18世纪中期在西欧大部分地区和美洲，接种都成为普遍做法。18世纪后半叶，接种方法的改进，以及给整个村子和城镇而不仅仅是个体接种，对公共卫生产生了越来越大的影响。伦敦这样的大城市比农村城镇更难以实现所有居民的接种，因此伦敦人仍继续遭受天花的袭击。接种改变了人们看待天花的方式：它成了一种有专门有效的方法来对抗的疾病。这为医疗史上最重要的突破——疫苗的出现铺平了道路。

1796年，爱德华·詹纳用少量牛痘代替人痘给一个英国小男孩接种来预防天花，这标志着消灭天花的曙光的出现。["疫苗"（vaccine）这个词也是詹纳发明的，他把牛痘称为牛天花（拉丁名 *variolae vaccinae*）。] 两年后他向全世界公布了他的发现。尽管在他之前也有人用牛痘给人接种，他的创新在于**证明**了这种方式是通过使人感染天花并获得免疫力而起效的。用减毒牛痘代替人痘接种很快就传播开来：它没有感染天花的危险，因此也没有播散的风险。詹纳公布牛痘接种方法后三年内有10万英国人接种了疫苗。之后二十年里又有几百万人接种：俄国有200万，法国也接近200万。1800年疫苗接种传到了北美；来年传到了巴格达，随后又传往印度。到19世纪中期，天花对北美印第安人的危害得到了遏制。牛痘接种（以及之前的人痘接种）减少了死亡人数。到1830年代，哈德逊湾公司给大部分加拿大西部的土著接种了疫苗；1770年代，危地马拉的殖民地医生开始给玛雅人接种，他们甚至采用了玛雅医疗技术，比如使用黑曜石刀。美洲的印第安人没有大规模地接种，开始接种的时机也很晚——这才造成了密苏里河沿岸的惨烈疫情。即便如此，因为越来越多的人有了免疫力，天花也不再被频繁引入，死亡人数也减少了。

作为一个曾经"闭关锁国"的国家，疫苗刚引入日本时受到了人们的怀疑乃至攻击。进口疫苗之士是促成日本向西方开放的先锋人物；疫苗是通往现代化的主要通道。1850年代，疫苗开始被人们所接受。德川幕府试图通过政府资助的疫苗接种项目把阿伊努人变得不那么"原始"，而更像日本人。该项目是否取得了成功没有定论。不过可以确定的是，疫苗出现后，阿伊努人长期以来对治愈天花的信念无法继续维系。疫苗这种有效新技术的出现使得整个信仰体系失效了。在欧洲，尽管早期出现了认为接种不卫生，或是怀疑能被另一种病毒所阻断的病原体是否存在之类的反对声音，但疫苗的应用仍然推广开来，特别是接种在有些地区成为强制措施。1800年瑞士有1.2万人死于天花。1822年减少到11人。随着天花所导致的死亡率的下降，欧洲人口开始增长。

尽管疫苗的使用早期取得了极大成功，但仍然出现了几次大规模的天花流行，因为疫苗使得天花发病率大大减少后，人们积极对抗疾病的热忱冷却下来，疫苗的效果也开始减退：疫苗并不能使人终身免疫，不过一开始无人知晓。1836—1839年英国有3万人死于天花。1870—1875年的天花大流行——由普法战争所引发——夺去了约50万人的生命，这使欧洲多国恢复了警惕。英国和德国通过了强制免疫法。不过在英国国内，对病因——环境、传染或瘴气导致——的争论，对政府强迫接种侵犯了公民身体的强烈不满，加上认为天花的重要性已经降低的观念，使得人们对强制免疫产生了激烈甚至暴力的反抗。1885年《接种法案》中的许多条款在1898年和1907年都被推翻。

尽管疫苗的使用使得人们放松了警惕，局部也频繁地有天

花疫情暴发，1870—1875年的欧洲天花大流行仍成为欧洲大陆上最后一次大规模的疫情。疫苗的使用以及重型天花慢慢被传染性更弱、症状更轻的轻型天花所代替，意味着到20世纪中期，天花在欧洲、美国和大多数发达国家都不再是重要的疾病。1971年美国公共卫生部建议取消常规接种，相比天花本身，当时有更多孩子——每年6～8个死于疫苗相关并发症。

天花疫苗的出现是公共卫生取得的巨大成就。它是针对个体健康的干预措施，并且对公众健康有着深远影响。使人群中易感者的数量减少以致传染性疾病无法传播，这是控制疾病的关键。而鼠疫期间采用的隔离等针对公共健康的早期措施则大不相同。隔离是为了在特定疫情期间阻止疫病的传播；疫苗从源头上降低疫病暴发的可能性。一旦足够数量的人都接种疫苗，找不到人类宿主的天花病毒就无处可去。

天花是唯一被人类根除的传染性疾病。最后一例重型天花于1975年发生在孟加拉；两年后最后一例轻型天花在索马里出现。1967年人们开展了大力清除天花的活动——起初世界卫生组织并不想对天花宣战，而是想消灭疟疾，不过以失败告终——十多年后世卫组织于1980年宣布人类已经消灭了天花。从任何方面来看——资金、物流、政治和社会层面的障碍、人道主义影响——消灭天花都是伟大的成就。

天花是传染性疾病中唯一理想的消灭对象。1940年代人们发明了冻干疫苗，这意味着理论上给热带地区居民接种这一难题已经被攻克。明显的脓疱使得天花很容易被辨认出来。1970年代早期，世卫组织的根除天花项目率先使用了隔离和疫病监测措施，这些举措取得了良好效果，阻止了疫病传播。天花再没

大
流
行
病

有动物宿主。不像由蚊子传播的疟疾,根除天花不需要考虑传播媒介,也不需要大规模的环境治理。根除天花的努力得到了国际社会的支持,世卫组织也因此投入了更多精力——在1967年变得声势浩大之前,根除天花没有多少实际行动;它只不过是41世卫组织一个不成熟的项目,人手不足,资金短缺。

为什么要根除天花?自从詹纳发明了疫苗,天花的发病率不断下降。尽管有些国家还有天花病例,但在大部分国家,天花已经不再是最急迫的公共卫生问题。更多地关注天花反倒减少了对疾病发病率增加原因的关注。在还有散发天花病例的地区比如拉丁美洲的许多国家,有人认为根除运动并不必要,它分散了对更严重的公共卫生问题的注意,而且耗资巨大。美国一国就投入了相当于现今10亿美元的资金到该项目中。不过资金主要来自开展根除运动的国家。在天花最猖獗的国家,比如非洲和南亚一些地区,每年仍然有200万人因此死亡。

根除天花的活动开展之后取得了快速的进展。几年的时间仍有天花流行的国家就减少到了四个——印度、孟加拉、巴基斯坦和埃塞俄比亚。印度的天花最顽固,世卫组织在此展开了最大规模的根除天花运动。在印度,哪怕根除运动并非一帆风顺并且伴随着冲突,但仍然进展迅速。因根除运动与英迪拉·甘地的独裁政府联手而产生的强制和威胁行为;印度当局和世卫组织以及地方官员和印度政府的分歧;疫苗供应和质量问题:所有这些以及其他更多困难使得印度的根除运动格外艰难。尽管如此,1975年印度仍然成功消灭了天花。

天花根除运动是成功的,但它不应被看作日内瓦发起的自上而下设计好的项目。根除运动实施的过程中,数不清的当地42

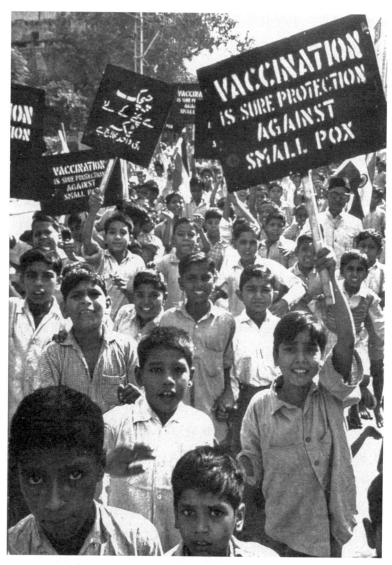

图3　印度儿童声援世卫组织和印度政府1950年代发起的根除天花运动。
43　公众对该项目的支持是成功的关键

人付出了辛劳,这对运动取得成功必不可少;频繁举办的国际会议促进了合作和经验分享,让人们从防控成功和失败的种种措施中学习。如果我们将根除运动的成功完全看作少数英雄人物运筹帷幄取得的战绩或世卫组织的功劳,那会伤害所有参与其中的人。这将是虚假的历史经验,会掩盖根除运动的本质:根除运动是对复杂的当地情况的应对,包含了多个层面、国际和当地人们的共同努力。简单化的陈述对任何人都没有好处。

活体天花病毒现在只存在于机密实验室中,在冷战期间它被美国和前苏联藏匿了起来。但在2014年6月,人们在美国国立卫生研究院的废弃仓库里发现了两瓶被遗忘数十年的活体天花病毒DNA。这一发现让人们短暂地回想起了天花这种曾令人畏惧的烈性传染病。

第三章

疟　疾

　　疟疾起源于非洲，是由疟原虫属（*Plasmodium*）的寄生性原生动物引起的。历史上大部分时期，人类感染过四种疟原虫：恶性疟原虫、三日疟原虫、卵形疟原虫和间日疟原虫。近来在东南亚因为砍伐森林，人类和灵长目动物的接触越来越频繁，由诺氏疟原虫（*P. knowlesi*）导致的疟疾日益增多。几种当中最常见的是恶性疟原虫和间日疟原虫。恶性疟原虫最凶险。全球由疟疾致死的病例中绝大多数是由恶性疟原虫引起的。

　　生活在500万年前的人类祖先可能就得过疟疾。但由于疟原虫的生命周期很复杂，需要满足一系列条件使大量蚊子和人类宿主同时存在才能形成流行。而且因为宿主常因为感染而死，疟原虫无法在体内长期存活——它和结核杆菌不同，后者感染人体后能终身潜伏——疟疾需要源源不断的新宿主。人口稠密是它传播的必要条件，而在距今1万年到4 000年前人类开始砍伐非洲中部的森林用于农业种植后，人口才慢慢开始变得密集。另外还需要数量庞大的蚊子。蚊子需要特定的生长环境：农民砍伐植被，清理吸水性良好的土地，由此形成了适合蚊子繁殖的水洼。因为能作为宿主的牲畜很少，按蚊（*Anopheles gamibiiac*）等蚊类开始吸食人血。当出现过疟疾疫情的人群与未感染过的缺乏免疫力的人群相遇时，疟疾才能传播开。 45

人们对疟疾在非洲以外地区的早期传播史知之甚少。公元前首个千年后，农业和人类活动导致环境变化，疟疾也随之出现，世界各地都发现了疟疾存在的确凿证据。罗马共和国晚期，经济形势迫使农民放弃了低洼耕地，随后这些耕地开始蓄水，变成疟疾横行的沼泽地带，罗马周围的地区也出现了疟疾疫情。砍伐森林以及曾运转良好的排水系统的年久失修使情况变得更糟。从那时起直到20世纪中期，意大利南部一直是疟疾在欧洲的据点。

疟疾随着农业发展在早期现代欧洲播散开来。15世纪晚期到19世纪中期大西洋奴隶贸易期间，它继续开疆拓土。17世纪和18世纪奴隶贸易最鼎盛的时期，热带非洲的疟疾抵达美洲热带地区。

和结核一样，疟疾的蔓延也离不开人对环境的塑造。城市环境导致了结核的出现，而农村和农业生产为疟疾铺平了道路。城市中心的扩张和农业生产密切相关：城市规模增长促进了农业发展。16世纪和17世纪的英格兰就是很好的例证，其人口增长和城市化进程使得农业生产更密集。在英格兰东南部的沼泽地带，为了发展农业，人们抽水排涝而把另一些地方变成了沼泽——这为蚊子的生存和疟疾蔓延创造了完美条件。持续拥入的农民提供了大量易感的人类宿主，疟疾因此传播开来。 46

国家之间的农业生产水平存在差异。通常在资本密集型农业得到发展的地区——美国和西欧等发达国家——农业就变得更加发达。在英国国内，这意味着更加先进的排水技术的出现和农村人口往城市的迁徙，人口的迁徙使得可能感染和传播疟疾的人也减少了。在发展中国家，农业没有得到普遍发展，仍然存在适合疟疾蔓延的条件以及易感人群。

通常来说，农业的进步和农村的发展是疟疾蔓延的原因，不过糟糕的城市卫生环境和不流动的水体会使疟疾在城市中传播——这种情况在发展中国家的大都市里越来越常见。另外，一些人造环境也促进了疟疾的产生。20世纪早期在巴拿马运河区，传播疟疾的主要是白魔按蚊（*A. albimanus*），运河的修建为它的繁殖创造了完美条件。当时一位昆虫学家写道："白魔按蚊和人关系密切，人的住所周围，人进行农业生产、工程建造和其他活动过程中营造的条件为它提供了最适宜的生存环境。"《巴拿马的蚊虫防治》（1916）的作者约瑟夫·勒普兰斯和A.J.奥伦斯坦写道，"大型挖掘和填埋施工中翻动了泥土，加上没有免疫力的工人住在工地附近"，这种情况下疟疾"传播得最快"。

随着农业定居和奴隶贸易的展开，从切诺皮克到密西西比流域，到加勒比海再到南美洲，疟疾都造成了惨重的伤亡。疟疾抵达美洲的确切日期无从知晓——或许它是随着早期英国移民从英国南部抵达切诺皮克的。17世纪中期，非洲黑奴带来了恶性疟疾。生活在美洲热带地区的移民和契约用人没有免疫力，疟疾在他们中间肆虐。人们发现黑人奴隶似乎不容易感染，便用黑奴取代了作为契约用人的欧洲人。奴隶贸易不仅给美洲带来了奴隶，也把非洲流行病区搬到了美洲。

就像面对19世纪的霍乱和早前的鼠疫一样，18世纪热带的

47

医生疑惑疾病究竟是地域的产物，还是它也会传播。其中的许多问题和种族及奴隶制度交织在了一起。看到不同种族死亡率的差异，许多人怀疑欧洲人是否注定会因为疟疾而死，而非洲奴隶一直都有抵抗力。这个问题令人困惑。正如1811年岁伯特·柯林斯博士在关于疟疾和黄热病的著作《甘蔗种植殖民地奴隶管理实用规则》中所写的："为什么黑人在疫病最严重的季节、最恶劣的条件下都安然无恙，而白人却大量死去？这一问题至今无人试着解答。"有人提出欧洲人将来会适应。在讨论这一主题的经典文章《热带气候下欧洲人易患病分析》（1786）中，詹姆斯·林德写道："随着时间的流逝，欧洲人的体质慢慢适应了东印度和西印度的气候……习惯之后，国外的欧洲人就和国内的欧洲人一样不大会得病。"这是否意味着可能所有的种族都能适应身边的环境和疾病？环境是否会决定生物学特性？18世纪许多人对这些问题的答案都是肯定的。

从19世纪开始，人们对种族的看法开始改变，气候影响健康而人会适应环境的观点慢慢消亡。种族被看作不同民族之间固有的坚不可摧的分界，欧洲人对于可以扎根热带的乐观看法被关于热带地区和"热带种族"的僵化观点所替代。就这样，热 48 带疟疾对医学的种族主义倾向起到了推波助澜的作用。

自17世纪热带地区出现疟疾以来，因为各种人类迁徙的影响，疟疾不断向内陆蔓延。在美国，农业种植和疟疾的前沿向西扩展到了俄亥俄州和密西西比流域。在巴西，金矿开采吸引人们前往内陆地区，疟疾也相伴而行。大规模的森林砍伐紧随其后，为建造大型农场让路，以便给大量劳工提供食物——在所谓的18世纪淘金世纪期间，有100多万非洲奴隶抵达内陆地区。

这为恶性疟疾的传播媒介达氏按蚊（*Anopheles darling*）创造了完美的栖息地，埋头工作的矿工则是完美的宿主。疟疾在人群当中大面积暴发。然而尽管直到20世纪疟疾仍然在美洲南部为患，英国的模式却一再重演：农业发展所带来的住房条件和营养状况改善，以及人类与蚊子接触减少，使得疟疾有所减轻。但在热带地区疟疾愈演愈烈，成为这些地区"合理"的一部分。

19世纪大部分时间里，疟疾和霍乱一样，都是典型的由腐烂剩菜和动物尸体所散发的瘴气而引发的疾病；雨水、种植及城市建设等翻动泥土的因素会引发瘴气的释放。疾病的名称甚至就意味着污浊的空气。病菌学说改变了这一切。1880年，阿方斯·拉韦朗在血液中发现了疟原虫，病理学技术的发展使得越来越多人亲眼看见并接受疟疾是由疟原虫引起的，瘴气理论渐渐式微。接着是传播媒介的发现。1898年，印度的罗纳德·罗斯和意大利的乔万尼·格拉西证明了按蚊会传播疟疾。疟疾的病因就与早前的霍乱和结核以及稍后的鼠疫一样，不再有各种各样而只有唯一的解释——感染疟原虫的蚊子的叮咬。带来的影响就是：控制传播媒介和疟原虫而非改善社会或经济条件，成为疟疾防治的主要方法。

在投入大量资源对蚊子发起不懈攻击，并且疟疾本来就不严重的地区，控制传播媒介的方法起效了。20世纪初在巴拿马运河区，美国负责改善地区卫生健康状况的威廉·戈加斯上校以前所未有的热情向疟疾和黄热病宣战，他努力研究掌握蚊子的繁殖习性和地点，再将它们消灭。美国充足的财力人力促成了这一切。两年之内黄热病就销声匿迹。消灭疟疾的时间更长——因为患过疟疾的人可能再次感染（相反，得过黄热病的人可以终身免疫），潜在的感染人群更庞大。不过疟疾最终败下阵来。

戈加斯的成功是公共卫生领域的成就，人们将其看作定居热带地区开启文明生活的重要步骤。1909 年《美国医学会杂志》上发表的题为《为白人征服热带地区》的文章中，戈加斯称他和同事们在巴拿马取得的成就是"白人能很好地在热带生活的最早例证，是白人真正定居热带的起点"。热带地区不适合白种人这一在 19 世纪占主流的观点被这种乐观看法推翻了。

使疟疾控制成为可能的发现催生了新的医疗研究领域——热带医学，它是致力于研究寄生虫及其传播媒介的科学。疟疾研究引领了这一学科的发展。正如热带医学的奠基人帕特里克·曼森所说，疟疾是"迄今为止……热带病理学上最重要的疾病"，因为它是"热带和亚热带地区主要的致病和致死原因"。这一新的研究领域衍生出培训项目、期刊和研究日程。欧洲和美国各地都设立了热带医学学院——利物浦热带医学学院成立最早，于 1987 年开放。疟疾防治的突破性进展和不断增加的对现代医学能够战胜疾病的信心，使得人们产生了强烈的乐观和自大情绪，也促进了热带医学这一学科的诞生。疟疾防控迫在眉睫，因为在许多地方，由于发展不平衡，疟疾仍在大规模流行，并且愈演愈烈。

农业的发展使得蚊子栖息地减少，生活质量提高意味着与疟疾接触机会减少，在这些地区疟疾的发病率有所下降。但在全球许多地区，历史上农民患病概率很高且无从逃避，现在仍然如此。在以农民为基础、投入不足的农业模式下，农民收入微薄，一直有染病的风险。主要种植单一作物、雇用农村贫困人口的大规模种植业通常为疟疾的播散创造了条件：砍伐森林用于耕种给蚊子创造了理想的繁殖地。由于大规模种植需要大量劳动力——在当地并不是总能找到——农村流动劳动力市场应运而生。就像大西洋奴隶贸易中，奴隶被迫迁徙将疟疾带往新大陆热带地区一样，19世纪和20世纪，非洲、南美洲和亚洲一些地区的劳动力迁徙也将疟疾传播到本来没有疟疾的地区，因为从无疟疾地区招收的工人返乡时将疾病一同带回了家乡。按照C.A.本特利和S.R.克里斯托弗斯在著作《杜阿尔斯地区的黑尿热病因》中的说法，从1860年代开始，"热带地区采用"以灌溉为基础的大规模农业模式使得疟疾成为印度的流行病。土壤排水差的地方，灌溉沟渠变成了一潭潭死水，为蚊子繁殖提供了理想条件；而大型茶叶种植园吸纳了大量的流动劳动力。这种情况非常利于流行性疟疾的传播。

　　历史上不同时期，劳动力的迁徙在许多地方引发了疟疾流行。例如，在巴西半干旱地区——大部分都没有疟疾疫情——因为苦于旱灾和佃农制度剥削，农民前往沿海地带和亚马孙雨林谋生。在工作的地方他们感染了疟疾，并且把疾病带回家乡，引起疟疾暴发。1936年，一场大面积的干旱迫使越来越多的人离乡背井，到外地工作。在沿海地带，他们遭遇了由冈比亚按蚊（*A. gambiae*）传播的烈性疟疾，这种蚊子是新近意外地随着西非船只抵达沿海的。沿海疫情的幸存者和来自疟疾更猖獗的亚马孙雨林的劳工一起回到干旱地区，引发了严重的疟疾疫情。这次疫情造成的死亡惨重：官方统计有五万人，实际可能更多。新闻报道中说，"语言无法描述这些地区的凄凉景象……人们都认为疫情之后东北地区将人烟稀少，因为那些侥幸逃生的人都会远走他乡"。

冈比亚按蚊的到来，以及因为社会经济因素被迫迁徙的大量易感者，共同造成了这次疫情。与之相似，1920年代和1930年代南非黑人被迫从没有疟疾的高地草原地区迁往疟疾泛滥的低地草原，也成为疟疾的潜在感染者。等他们回到侵占土地的人所经营的种植园时，他们也带回了疟疾。相似的情况在热带地区越来越普遍，丝毫没有停止的迹象，人们必须找到一个解决办法。

有志控制疟疾的人士因为支持的方法不同而分成了两个阵营：灭蚊或是治疗疟原虫感染。戈加斯在巴拿马和古巴的成功经验激起了人们对消灭传播媒介的信心，而奎宁的发明使得治疗疟原虫感染成为可能。两种方法各有其优缺点。奎宁的预防效果有限，但它的治疗作用弥补了这一不足。它可以缓解症状，不过供应可能不稳定，而且大规模使用起来成本高昂；奎宁很难吃，人们不容易接受。另外，奎宁不能阻止疟疾的传播，也就是说感染疟原虫的病人可以用奎宁减轻症状，但是他们还会传播疾病。控制传播媒介的方法也有效。它的缺点在于花费巨大而且物流很复杂，许多地方无法获得足够的资源。两种方法都没有触及疟疾之所以长期存在的深层原因。

控制传播媒介的方法在许多地区大获成功，渐渐成为主流。戈加斯或许是这一方法的开创者，不过还有许多成功控制媒介的方法，比如改善按蚊繁殖地环境的卫生策略。这种方法由马来西亚的马尔科姆·沃森发起，第一次世界大战前由N.R.斯韦伦格列伯加以改良，随后大获成功。1920年代和1930年代在意大利，墨索里尼的法西斯政府抽干了蓬蒂内沼泽，把它重新变成农田，并且让人们在此定居，从而控制了疟疾疫情。在巴勒斯坦，小规模的农业改良和媒介控制遏制了疟疾的势头。在大萧条时期的美国，田纳西河流域管理局发起了消灭疟疾的农业改良运动。降低蓄水库的水位让按蚊卵脱水，为门窗加纱窗（19世纪后这种做法越来越普遍），在蚊子繁殖地带喷洒杀灭幼虫的药，以及在河岸开辟放牧区为蚊子提供宿主等等，所有这些措施让美国南部的疟疾发病率持续下降。

　　第二次世界大战前后包括二战期间，控制媒介作为防治疟疾主要措施的地位得到了巩固。人们在按蚊生态学上取得了突破，特别是对携带和不携带疟疾的蚊子种类了解越来越深入；弗莱德·索珀和洛克菲勒基金会在消灭巴西的冈比亚按蚊上取得了成功；第二次世界大战期间杀虫剂DDT的发明；以及战后促使各国接连向结核宣战的同样的热情：所有这一切促成了媒介控制的成功。疟疾、结核还有天花一道成为刚成立的世界卫生组织战后全球卫生项目的防控目标。

　　消灭疟疾是和全球推进民主与资本主义紧密联系在一起的。1956年美国国际发展局宣称，疟疾防治减轻了爪哇城市人口拥挤的现状，并且促使越盟控制地区向喷洒DDT的团队开放，消灭菲律宾农村的疟疾意味着原本没有地的农民可以在新回收的土地上耕种——以免他们沦为"胡克"①（Huk）武装成员。控制疟疾就意味着传播民主。"疟疾阻碍社会发展"——疟疾决定了是成为经济发达的现代化国家，还是深陷传统桎梏和贫困当中——这种看法很普遍。疟疾防控专家保罗·拉塞尔说得很清楚：疟疾使得"国家容易受到政治病菌的毒害，阻碍并且摧毁自由"。有些人比如美国结核病专家沃尔什·麦克德莫特

---

　　① 菲律宾人民抗日军。——编注

就认为，生物医学是成为现代化国家的关键。"全球发展过程中生物医学的目标，或者说是有目的地实现现代化，就是改变一个极度传统社会的疾病模式，使其不会成为现代化的主要阻碍。"

控制疟疾的乐观情绪空前高涨，世卫组织决心根除疟疾。就像疟疾成为热带疾病的代表一样，它也成了充斥着自大和过分乐观情绪的时代的象征。大量医学成就的取得特别是抗生素和DDT的发明，让人们开始畅想消灭某些疾病的时代已经来临。正是在这样的背景下，传染病专家T.艾丹·科伯恩1961年在《科学》杂志中写道："我们有信心在不久的将来，人类将在很大程度上摆脱传染性疾病。"

疟疾很自然地成了根除的目标。人们对蚊子的繁殖规律和哪些种类会传播疟疾的了解越来越深入，有巴西成功消灭疟疾的经验在先，而且拥有了专门灭蚊的药物，这些因素共同促进了战后消灭疟疾运动向发展中国家的强势推进，人们向疟疾发动了史无前例的战争。另外很重要的一点是，1955年世卫组织正式宣布消灭疟疾项目启动时，全球卫生官僚系统规模比如今小得多：专家的数量相对较少；许多专家的意见一致；大部分都是世卫组织疟疾专家委员会的成员。一个规模很小的专家团队决定采用室内滞留性喷洒DDT的方式消灭疟疾。起主导作用的是世卫组织和美国等出资国政府，联合国儿童基金会发挥重要的协同作用。项目资金主要来自美国和联合国儿童基金会等联合国机构，当地政府负责剩余的部分——常常花费巨大而收效甚微。

事件的进展表明世卫组织对消灭疟疾项目的信心是盲目的。14年的消灭疟疾运动表明，疟疾在实践中比理论上要难消灭得多。早期根除运动在委内瑞拉等国取得了成功，十年后就举步维艰。尽管大部分疟疾病例都在非洲，但除了开展一些示范项目，世卫组织根本就没试过要消灭非洲的疟疾。非洲的基础设施太薄弱，疟疾太严重；根除疟疾在非洲是不可能的。因此没有人去尝试。而在印度，国家体量庞大，项目人员臃肿多达15万，大部分地区缺乏基本医疗，而DDT的抗药性问题越来越突出，这一切使得人们得出了无法在印度根除疟疾的结论。

在巴西等其他国家，主张根除疟疾者的激进观点和现行的疟疾控制项目起了冲突，但世卫组织、泛美卫生组织的卫生部门领导和最大的资助者美国仍然支持根除。巴西和墨西哥几乎是被迫接受了根除项目，项目起初取得了成功，之后遭遇失败。根除项目终止后，蚊子（不可避免地）卷土重来，当地的人们几乎没有免疫力，防蚊项目也取消了。随后又出现了耐药性问题：首先，到1969年56种蚊子已经对DDT产生了耐药性；其次，由于不负责任地大规模用药，耐药蚊子引发的疟疾对奎宁也有了抗性。

消灭疟疾项目还是取得了一些成功。参与项目的国家中有39%消灭了疟疾，部分加勒比海地区和东欧国家不再有疟疾的身影。尽管如此，当1969年世卫组织意识到消灭疟疾活动并未起效时，仍然终止了这个项目。过度关注单一的技术性解决方案而忽视了疟疾的政治经济因素；人们对DDT的安全性越来越担忧，特别是在蕾切尔·卡森《寂静的春天》出版后；杀虫药和治疗疟疾药物的耐药性问题；资金来源不稳定：这些都导致了这一项目的失败。

1960年代开始，疟疾以惊人的势头卷土重来。在印度和巴

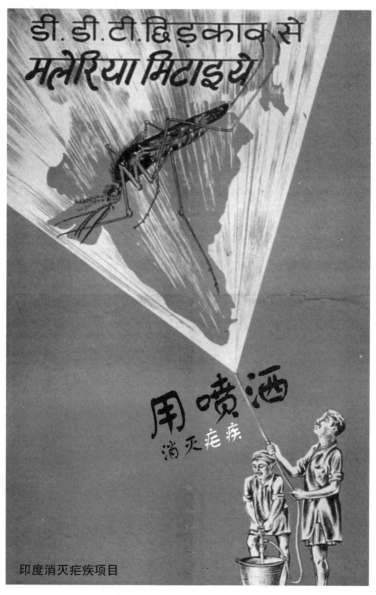

印度消灭疟疾项目

图4 1950年代，在世界范围内，通过发行纪念邮票、张贴海报（如图）、无线电广播节目和其他方式，世卫组织的消灭疟疾运动得到了大张旗鼓的宣传

56

西等疟疾防治取得显著成效的国家,疟疾又重新抬头。1960年代初印度只有不到10万疟疾病例,到1965年就增长到原来的1.5倍,这主要是卫生设施薄弱的各邦监控和后续行动不利引起的;DDT供应不稳定还有耐药性都加剧了这一问题。而在疟疾从未被真正压制住的非洲,情况进一步恶化。在赞比亚和斯威士兰,农业发展、艾滋病、贫困加剧以及杀虫剂和抗疟药作用减弱都使得疟疾发病率出现上升。人口流动增加和卫生设施老旧也使得情况雪上加霜。全球经济发展模式促进了经济发展不平等加剧和大规模债务产生,使得用于疟疾防治(和其他疾病)的资金减少。

为了应对卷土重来的疟疾,全球发起了另一项控制疟疾的运动——1998年由世界银行赞助的"遏制疟疾"项目。遏制疟疾项目和抗艾滋病、结核和疟疾全球基金唤起了人们对疟疾的关注,吸引了更多资助。然而疟疾发病率仍然不断增加。尽管该项目的目标不是根除疟疾,也将非洲纳入了项目当中,但它在一些关键问题上和根除项目有相似之处:它没有考虑疟疾再次抬头的原因;项目开展当地基础卫生设施薄弱;控制疟疾没有相应地发展经济;没有考虑项目开展地的实际情况。尽管杀虫剂处理过的蚊帐作为主要措施在许多地方都发挥了巨大的作用——世卫组织声称自2000年以来蚊帐已经使得非洲的疟疾感染率下降了一半——但在尼日利亚、莫桑比克等地大量蚊帐被人们改成了渔网。在捕鱼填饱肚子和蚊帐防蚊之间,几百万人都选择了填饱肚子。捕鱼活动增加使得鱼的数量下降。蚊帐本来是用来控制疟疾的,现在却变成了谋生工具,在这个过程中产生的过度捕捞又威胁到了人们赖以为生的食物来源。

这些项目都没有考虑促使疟疾发病率增加的环境条件。盖茨基金会把大部分资金都投入到疫苗研发当中，同时基金会再度唤起了人们对根除疟疾的兴趣。2015年5月的世界卫生大会上，世卫组织再次承诺要根除疟疾。不管全世界多么希望消灭疟疾，只关注一种疾病必然会带来一些后果。在赞比亚等疟疾呈上升态势的国家，尽管控制疟疾的努力收到了成效，但最近有人指出这是以牺牲其他的卫生措施为代价的。只关注疟疾这样单一的疾病会夺走其他注重改善整体健康状况的项目的资源。

控制疟疾的最大挑战之一是耐药性。从抗疟药和杀虫剂问世之初就存在耐药性的困扰，人们的忽视和对其他更紧迫的问题的关注使得这一问题越发严重。如今，一直以来最有效的抗疟药青蒿素的效果日益减退。21世纪初，柬埔寨出现了对青蒿素耐药的疟疾；2015年早些时候，耐药的恶性疟疾通过人和传播媒介的迁徙播散了1 500英里——抵达印缅交界地区。一旦耐青蒿素的疟疾传播到非洲，将会有灾难性的后果。

自19世纪末以来，找到根除疟疾的技术手段，不论是蚊帐或是更有效的药物，一直是疟疾控制的目标，也是控制疟疾的核心信条。这种做法的好处显而易见。20世纪中期，用技术消灭疟疾传播媒介的时机似乎已经成熟，和根除或改善助长疟疾的社会环境比起来，这个目标要容易得多。

59

第四章

霍 乱

霍乱是一种可怕的疾病，它是由饮用被带菌粪便污染过的水引起的。一旦感染霍乱弧菌（*Vibrio cholerae*），可怕的症状便很快出现——病人脸色苍白憔悴，形容枯槁，体液快速大量流失，往往会有生命危险。在几百年的时间里人们对它束手无策。1960年代，在孟加拉工作的医生和研究人员发现用糖盐水可以补充因为霍乱（以及几乎任何其他腹泻）丢失的体液。口服补液法因此挽救了数百万人的生命。

尽管自18世纪甚至更早以来印度一直就有霍乱病例，但1817年的霍乱因为影响范围广、情况严重，往往被看作霍乱作为大流行病的开端。自那时起世界范围内暴发了七次霍乱大流行，前六次都是所谓的"古典型霍乱"（*V. cholera* 01）。每次大流行最后都慢慢平息下来，只剩下南亚有少数病例。1923—1961年的整整38年间没有发生全球霍乱疫情。后来由于未知的原因，埃尔托生物型——按照发现地埃及的埃尔托命名——取代了古典型引发了第七次大流行并且持续至今。

和结核不同，霍乱不是人们熟知的常见病。在人们产生越来越强烈的憎恶和恐惧的异域东方，它无声无息地神秘降临了。60人们不知道它的病因，也不知道如何治疗。随着它在城市的穷人当中和来自印度及其他国家的移民之间泛滥开来，霍乱成为肮脏和落后的象征。霍乱暴露了人们的焦虑，反映出不同医学流派的深刻分歧，揭示了巴黎、伦敦、那不勒斯和汉堡等地的阶级和贫富分化。

　　虽然每次霍乱流行都有一些相同的主题——害怕、对病因和治疗方法的争论、霍乱的症状和危害在人群中引发的恐惧——但每次都有不同之处。1831—1832年英国的疫情比1848—1849年轻微得多，后者的死亡人数是前者的两倍，但人们

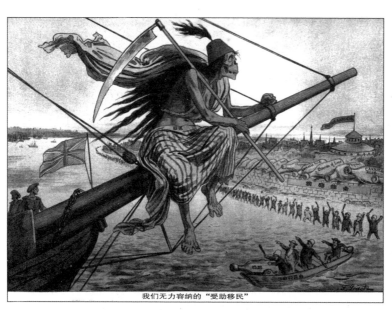

我们无力容纳的"受助移民"

图5　对外来者的恐惧在霍乱流行期间达到了顶峰。这幅1883年的漫画描绘了移民船携带着霍乱在美国海港靠岸的情景

的恐慌情绪更严重。第七次大流行——现在仍未结束——完全绕过了1911年之后就再也没有霍乱身影的欧洲。然而2010年
61 霍乱出现在海地,终结了那里一百多年没有疫情的历史。非洲直到1865—1871年第四次霍乱大流行前都没有出现过严重的霍乱疫情,现在的病例却是最多的。

在有些观察家看来,霍乱发生在某些国家而不是其他国家,反映出文明卫生和肮脏落后之间的本质区别。1833年,一位将霍乱看作来自印度的野蛮入侵的法国作家谈到霍乱流行时写道:"有理由相信,如果恒河两岸的居民有幸生活在民主政府的统治之下,他们一定可以控制疫病,而疫病正是恒河排出带病的有毒河水污染其他国家导致的。自由的力量可以从源头上击退瘟疫。"

霍乱象征着世界变得越来越小,国家的联系越来越紧密,疾病轻易就跨越了国界。参加1851年世界卫生大会的法国代表指出:

> 加上如今人们交往繁多,交往也越来越便利;人们可以乘坐蒸汽船和火车旅行,还有人们越来越乐于互相拜访、彼此融合,似乎要把不同的民族变成单一大家庭,你不得不承认在这样的情况下,对于霍乱这样一种传播广泛的疾病,封锁和隔离不但毫无效果,而且绝大多数时候是不可能的。

霍乱发源于何处? 1830年代早期,许多人认为它来自印度——明确地说是孟加拉——从更广泛的意义上说来自亚洲。近期对霍乱的生物史研究让答案不那么肯定——它的多变、和许多胃肠道疾病类似的临床表现、基因组不稳定性、能在世界各地海洋环境中存活的能力都表明,19世纪人们确认的亚洲霍乱

可能并不仅仅发源于亚洲。因此1817年以前欧洲的霍乱样流行病可能就是霍乱——19世纪那些认为霍乱只可能来自印度的人们对此不屑一顾。

把霍乱和印度联系在一起给这个国家打上了永久的耻辱印记。因为未知的原因——或许是出现了新的毒株；自霍乱在印度暴发可能已过去了几十年——1817年的霍乱毒性特别强，1819年东印度公司的两名医生称之为"现代以来印度发生的最可怕的致死性疾病"。尽管不同的估计数字之间有出入，但1817—1831年间疫病可能导致了几百万印度人死亡，其中大多数是营养不良的穷苦农民。霍乱在整个印度大陆肆虐，但孟加拉是疫情最严重的地区。

霍乱不仅仅是差异或是联系紧密的世界的象征。它是真实的存在。1831年欧洲突如其来的霍乱疫情让人们惊慌失措，在有些人看来这意味着另一场鼠疫。有人像鼠疫流行期间一样外逃躲避，有人留守下来。对霍乱的恐惧有时和实际危险并不相符。1831年，霍乱途经俄国造访英国时，紧张不安的人们等待着它的降临。报纸、宣传单和流言散播着对疾病的恐慌。《医学外科评论》的编辑詹姆斯·约翰逊博士在给《泰晤士报》的一封信中提醒媒体："毫无疑问，对霍乱的恐慌就像疾病一样正在英国各处肆虐……被这种情绪惊吓而死的人将比霍乱本身造成的伤亡人数多得多。"

目睹了霍乱在途经俄国播散到英国途中造成的惨重伤亡，一位惊慌失措的作家在《评论季刊》上写道：

> 如今我们目睹了一场新瘟疫的降临，它在短短14年的

时间里播散到世界各地，夺走了至少 5 000 万人的性命。它适应了各种气候，跨越了种种天然屏障，征服了每一个民族。它不像沙尘暴，在造成破坏后就消失无踪；它和天花或鼠疫一样，会在占领过的地方扎下根来。

1832 年，英国有一些地方爆发了骚乱。当时几起盗墓案被媒体广泛报道，还有一起骇人听闻、谈论得沸沸扬扬的为尸害命案件，暴徒们怀疑医生为了给医学院的解剖课收集尸体而毒害穷人，从而把怒火发泄到医生身上。在法国，人们担心富人利用霍乱除掉穷人。霍乱对西方人在生物学和文化上的优越感提出了质疑：来自原始落后的东方的疾病怎么会让现代进步的西方陷入瘫痪呢？霍乱暴露出快速工业化进程中涌现出的欧洲大都市里可怕的生存状况。让欧洲变得现代化的因素会不会也是引发霍乱的元凶呢？

不管是否必要，恐慌情绪会带来严重的后果。1911 年那不勒斯发生了霍乱，意大利政府极度担心疫情可能的影响——贸易和旅游活动会受到影响甚至中断；移民受限；人们将认为意大利不是现代、卫生的国家——以至于对外隐瞒了疫情的消息。

有一些关于霍乱的未解之谜特别重要，人们花了 19 世纪大部分的时间来试图解开它们，同时这些谜题也不仅限于霍乱。因为不是人人都同样得病，人们奇怪为什么有人会感染而其他人却不会。它会不会传染，就像 1830 年代人们认为有传染性的天花和鼠疫一样？它是由瘴气导致的吗？它是天花和鼠疫这两种病的结合吗？支持传染学说一般意味着赞同隔离等措施。而瘴气理论的支持者认为隔离毫无效果；他们认为疾病是由臭气——腐烂的蔬菜和土壤中的动物尸体以及它们产生的浊气——的释放引发的。两种理论之间没有截然的分界。此外，因为选择某些而忽视其他事实在方法学上站不住脚，要提出病因的合理解释是很困难的；大多数人选择相信和理论相符的事实。一位作家在《柳叶刀》上总结说："作为一种归纳科学，医学的发展被提出假想理论，或者说无用和虚妄的假设原则，以及从少数事实推断出普遍原则或结论这种方法所拖累。"

虽然关于霍乱的传播途径有各种各样的解释——这种情况会持续几十年——但短期内人们必须采取措施。从这一点上看几乎人人都是传染学说支持者：不管是英法等民主国家，还是俄国、奥匈帝国、普鲁士等独裁国家，政府最初的应对方法都是依照抗击鼠疫的历史经验来防治霍乱，施行隔离和旅行禁令。为了防止霍乱传播，政府重新施行防疫边界政策；详细标记病患和疑似感染者，必要的时候将他们隔离；封锁感染地区；积极清洁和消毒人员与货物。1830年秋霍乱袭击莫斯科之际，俄国采取了激进的防护措施——毁坏道路、破坏桥梁、封锁进出城的通路。军队实施了禁足令，违反者将被处决。在200英里长的东部国界上有六万军队驻守。面对这些严厉的措施，有人漠不关心，有人害怕，有人愤怒，有人反抗。在莫斯科和圣彼得堡，强制让病人住院的政策引发了大范围的抗议。在维捷格拉，满腔义愤的暴乱分子解救了被迫关押起来的病人并且破坏了医院里的设施。

专制政府不只采取了阻止传染相关的措施，他们还考虑实际情况，制定了基本的卫生策略——大部分是没有实际效力的关于改善卫生状况的劝诫——针对的主要是穷人。霍乱的发生

65

可能和本地的状况有关，患病的大多数是穷人，这都意味着它可能不仅仅是传染造成的。人们对霍乱的传播途径越来越不肯定，对日常生活的严格限制普遍不满，商人对隔离强烈反对，以及隔离对贸易的影响使得政府的态度发生了转变。随着政府、医生、大众和卫生官员应对霍乱的经验越来越丰富，早期的贸易和旅行禁令越来越难以实施。另外，不断增加的证据表明这些措施收效甚微，于是政府开始放宽限制。再加上霍乱沿着贸易通道向西传播的过程中，受影响的国家吸取了已经发生过疫情的国家的经验，比如俄国的经验就表明隔离措施没有效果。因此，1830年代中期，欧洲的第一次霍乱疫情平息下来的时候，人们对传染学说的支持开始下降。早期人们对霍乱的强烈恐惧再也没有重演。1840年代和1850年代霍乱再次袭来时，人们的反应大不一样，德国的吕贝克和汉堡采取了不作为的政策；和对霍乱的担忧相比，当局更担心贸易禁令和民众不满的后果。

不过在第一次霍乱冲击渐渐平息和疫情得到控制后，人们开始反思。依靠抗击鼠疫的历史经验来防治霍乱并不恰当，必须提出对病因的解释和其他的防控办法。霍乱是一种在人与人之间传播的传染病的观念被摒弃。霍乱是当地环境所造成的这种解释同样不能令人信服——在同一地方并非所有人都会染病。有人相信霍乱是上帝对懒惰和罪过的惩罚，是不道德的行为导致的。许多人注意到霍乱和贫穷两者的关联。居住环境或许可以部分解释霍乱为什么会危害特定的地方和人群。

贫穷和流行性疾病之间的关联不是在霍乱流行期间产生的，人们很早以前就将贫穷和鼠疫联系在一起。不过在1820年代和1830年代，人们更进一步探讨了两者的关系。1820年代，路易-勒内·维莱梅在巴黎进行的人口统计研究提出，巴黎最穷困地区居民健康状况不佳的原因是经济状况而非环境因素。英国人口学家威廉·法尔在英国城市中心发现了同样的关联。席卷欧洲的快速工业化和城市化进程导致贫困，促进了霍乱的发生。这一解释可以很好地迎合传染和瘴气理论。可能的情况是穷人居住在充满瘴气的环境里，非常适合感染性疾病霍乱的传播。霍乱病因的环境学说开始占主导地位。

　　这种观点在英国得到广泛传播，促使公共卫生领域产生了变革。对特定地区和霍乱（以及广泛意义上的疾病）存在关联这一理论最支持的是埃德温·查德威克，他于1830年担任制定《济贫法》的官员。他被贫穷和疾病相关这一理论所吸引，同时致力于践行哲学家杰里米·边沁的观点。查德威克和一些医生在1842年发表了《英国劳工卫生状况报告》，文中用大量的地图、图表和数据来说明疾病、贫穷和某些街区的卫生状况这三者的联系，成为英国卫生运动的依据。1848年《公共卫生法案》的通过和卫生总局的成立标志着卫生运动达到了高潮。维莱梅认为不公正的经济制度造成了严重的贫富差距；而查德威克作为忠实的瘴气理论支持者，眼中只有污秽和干净的环境。不需要进行大规模的社会经济改革，只需要改善城市环境就可以了。查德威克和支持者们主张建造供水和能随时冲走产生瘴气的垃圾的排水系统。查德威克的构想用了五十年的时间才完全实现，它将和巴黎的下水道系统一道成为19世纪伟大的工程成就。有了洁净的水居民自然会更健康，但对干净用水的呼吁并不总是甚至并不常是出于对穷人健康状况的担心，而更多是为了满足消费者和工厂的要求。

任何有心之士都很容易看出城市化、肮脏的居住环境和疾病的关联。和查德威克持有同样观点的人认为水可以冲走污染环境的瘴气和生活垃圾。他们没有想过可能问题在于水本身。但是约翰·斯诺想到了，1854年霍乱流行期间，他在伦敦开展了开创性的流行病学研究。在1848年霍乱流行期间，他就开始思考霍乱的来源，1849年发表了题为《霍乱传播途径探讨》的文章。他怀疑霍乱患者的粪便污染了水源。在他看来，霍乱和天花不同，不是通过空气在人群中传播的，因为霍乱不是肺部而是肠道疾病。霍乱通过水传播的理论在当时还只是一个猜测——不过斯诺很快就有机会来加以验证。

1854年霍乱流行期间，斯诺画出了所有霍乱病例的分布图，分析患者饮用的水来自何处，这成为流行病学的经典案例。结果明白无误：斯诺发现苏荷区所有患者喝的都是来自宽街水井的水。在斯诺成功说服政府取下了水泵把手后，霍乱病例骤减。结论很明确：水被污染了。但当时没人知道水中到底有什么。

1860年代，相信霍乱是一种传染病的观点渐渐占了上风，但仍然有人认为瘴气理论才能完美解释霍乱的成因。印度有人认为印度次大陆之所以饱受霍乱侵袭，是因为疾病潜藏在泥土中，靠空气传播，专门祸害那些容易感染的弱势群体。印度卫生官员相信隔离商船或是实行封锁来阻止霍乱传播，"就像用一队哨兵来阻挡季风一样不合常理也没有效果"。不过这些观点和医学发展的方向相抵触。

让瘴气理论真正消亡的是1883年第五次霍乱流行期间罗伯特·科赫在细菌学研究上取得的成就，尽管一开始这些成果没有引起很大反响。分离出炭疽和结核菌后，科赫开始研究霍

68

乱。科赫在被污染的水中发现了形似逗号的霍乱弧菌，得出是它引发霍乱的结论后，瘴气理论的末日也宣告到来了。

并非所有人都赞同科赫和斯诺的理论。改良版的瘴气学说仍然有一定影响。著名德国卫生学家马克斯·冯·佩腾科费尔继续要求政府提供洁净的饮用水，不是因为他相信霍乱是污染的水传播的，而是因为干净卫生是保持健康的关键。他认为垃圾腐败物污染地下水从而产生了霍乱。佩腾科费尔的观点在一段时期内深刻影响了德国政府的卫生政策，例如政府针对是否为汉堡最贫困的居民提供干净饮用水的决策就受其影响（他们没有提供净水）。1892年汉堡市暴发了霍乱，而附近有净水供应的阿尔托纳市却得以幸免，水源传播理论的支持者——至此大部分医学专家和相关人士都加入其中——被证明是正确的。然而佩腾科费尔仍然坚持他的观点。为此他喝下被霍乱弧菌污染的水，得了腹泻——不过据他自己说不是严重的霍乱。在他看来，没有局部具体的卫生和气候条件（Y因子），单独的X因子（霍乱弧菌）不足以形成局部流行（Z因子）。在他进行试验期间，他这样的观点已经渐渐失去了影响力。

随着海洋和陆地旅行越来越快捷，"文明"的西方与"落后"的东方以及东方疾病的接触越来越频繁，传染理论越来越深入人心。对疾病传播的担忧使得人们进入新式隔离政策、医学检疫、旅行禁令和医学国际主义大行其道的年代。此后，始于1850年代的国际卫生大会定期召开，各国齐聚一堂，商讨日益频繁的全球旅行和贸易相关问题。1865年霍乱疫情暴发，前往麦加朝圣的人群将霍乱播散开来，全球对流行病越来越关切。

在之前的疫情中，霍乱从印度传播到欧洲用了六年的时间。

铁路和蒸汽船把地中海和红海连通后，1865年的疫情只用了两年。1870年代，国际卫生大会成为讨论限制来自中东和印度旅客的论坛。1872年，意大利代表陈词："众所周知，我们要阻止该死的印度旅客，不让他上路，至少我们要在离他的出发地尽可能近的地方把他拦住。"不只印度，整个东方对西方来说都是威胁。正如1892年一位作家在《印度时报》上发表的文章中写到的："欧洲的真正威胁来自朝圣地麦加、阿拉伯人聚居区、卡尔巴拉、大马士革、耶路撒冷、波斯的不同城市以及朝圣者的碰头地点……因为苦修而身体虚弱的朝圣者成了病菌的目标，而朝圣地肮脏的环境和卫生政策缺乏或者说有效卫生政策的缺位促进了疾病的传播。"马克·哈里森将之称为"遏制东方"的政策。随着越来越激烈的全球竞争需要人员和货物的自由流动，意大利和英国等国家不再积极实行贸易和旅行禁令，对东方的遏制也缓和下来。与此同时，霍乱与东方特别是印度有关这种观点根深蒂固。

20世纪早期，在西欧和美国，霍乱某种程度上成为过去。1911年意大利暴发了霍乱，政府不遗余力地掩盖疫情正说明了在快速现代化的欧洲，霍乱是多么罕见和令人恐惧。1920年代，霍乱已经在发展中国家深深扎根，而发达国家也不再关注这种疾病。

第七次霍乱流行对非洲的打击最大——90%的霍乱病例发生在非洲。迈伦·埃琴伯格公正地指出，非洲的遭遇提出了一个问题：在人们对霍乱的了解越来越深入并且拥有便宜有效的治疗措施的情况下，霍乱为何愈演愈烈，夺去了更多人的性命？原因和结核与疟疾仍困扰着许多非洲地区的原因一样：1970年代以来，卫生设施的匮乏、越来越不稳定的经济状况、日益加剧的贫富差距、落后的卫生条件共同促进了霍乱的持续流行。战争带来的人口流动也加快了霍乱的传播。

第七次霍乱流行和前六次整体上有很明显的区别。它波及新的地区或长期以来没有疫情的地区，比如原苏联和拉丁美洲；它的传播速度很快；持续时间比前六次都长——猖獗的态势已经持续了四十年的时间，还没有消亡的迹象；埃尔托生物型比古典型毒力弱，因此也容易传播。

71

霍乱比任何其他传染病都更像是社会不公的产物和象征。在有稳定和干净的水供应的地方，霍乱就无法生存。气候变化可能会使情况变得更糟，霍乱将会传播到那些受海水温度升高（在这样的温度下霍乱弧菌会滋长）影响最大又无法使之减轻的国家。

72

结 核

结核分枝杆菌（*Mycobacterium tuberculosis*）引发的结核可能是人类最古老的一种疾病。结核分枝杆菌是分枝杆菌属的一员，其中包括非洲分枝杆菌（*M. africanum*）、牛分枝杆菌（*M. bovis*）和卡内蒂分枝杆菌（*M. cannetti*），它们可能已经演化了三亿年。土耳其发现的距今五十万年前的直立人头骨上的结核样病灶可能是最古老的结核病化石证据。感染人类的结核分枝杆菌大约七万年前出现在非洲。它和现代人类一同踏上了迁徙之旅，走出非洲，先是越过了印度洋，几千年后到达欧亚大陆。大约一万年前人类定居下来并且聚居在一起，结核就开始蔓延起来。在那之后结核从未消亡。

结核可以感染身体的几乎各个部位——骨骼、血液和大脑。其中最常见、最致命的是肺结核，它通过空气中的飞沫传播，传染性很强。人口密集的地方利于结核病的传播。

结核和鼠疫一样是一种古老的疾病，关于它的历史记载同样悠久。人们也曾经从传染和瘴气学说两方面讨论过其病因。

回顾性诊断难度很大，它的症状可能和肺炎或者其他肺部疾病
混淆。根据几百年来人们对结核症状的描述——盗汗、体重减
轻、干咳——来确诊很困难。结核病引发了疾病研究的实验室
变革，1882年罗伯特·科赫在显微镜下发现的正是导致结核的
分枝杆菌。过去人们眼中有着不确定但多种多样病因的消耗
性疾病和肺痨，变成了一种确切的由单一因素引发的疾病——
结核。

　　结核不像鼠疫会突然暴发，夺去几百万人的生命；它是一种
慢性疾病。没有人认为它是上帝发怒降罪到人间，惩罚罪人的。
它的症状也不像霍乱那样可怕。它不会一下子将人击垮，使人
呕吐大量体液后几小时内生命垂危。它是隐袭性的，一开始不
会被发现。它不像19世纪的霍乱一样激起媒体和公众的强烈
反应，也不像鼠疫使得人们因为恐慌残害同胞。然而结核导致
的死亡比这两种疾病都要多得多。早在17世纪，《死亡统计表》
（Bills of Mortality）——伦敦早期流行病学历史记录——就表
明，结核占伦敦居民死因的20%。

　　过去人们对结核的认知和现在大不相同。17世纪末理查
德·莫顿所著的《痨病学》（Phthisiologia）讨论了结核病的不同
形式，这本书先是用拉丁文出版，后来翻译成英文。例如，在莫
顿看来，吞指甲或是肺部被扎伤会导致结核，妇女产乳过多、耗
伤气血导致体虚和神情冷漠也会引发结核。尽管这听起来不像
现在我们知道的结核，但莫顿对肺部结核结节的描述和现代的
结核很相似。托马斯·西德纳姆认为最有效的治疗方式就是骑
马长途旅行。

　　18世纪对结核的描述越来越精确。意大利和英国的解剖

学家在身体几乎各个部位都发现了结核结节。18世纪早期，勒内·拉埃奈克统一了当时流传的对结节的病理性描述后，模糊的表述就慢慢消失了。他在书中写道，没有结节就没有结核病。他发明了可以探听身体内部各种声音的听诊器，正是有了听诊器才得出了这些结论。过去医生都是根据病人的讲述和自己对症状的观察来诊断结核，拉埃奈克专注于结节，他用听诊器来发现结节，死后通过尸检加以证实。从拉埃奈克的听诊器到科赫的显微镜有一条清晰的发展路径。在拉埃奈克和其他一些同样专注于研究致病性生物的巴黎医生之后，结核作为单一疾病受到广泛关注。1839年，瑞士医学教授 J. L. 舍恩莱因把所有有结节的病都归到结核之下，结核病正式得名。1882年科赫在显微镜下的发现证实了这一切。

尽管结核不像霍乱那样引发人们的恐慌和排外情绪，不过它仍然成了文学和歌剧的主题（最有名的要属威尔第的《波希米亚人》），而身患结核的浪漫诗人（首先想到的就是济慈）在19世纪的欧洲文学史上一度占有特殊的地位。那些常年不见阳光，宁愿整天待在室内、脸色惨白、精神萎靡的上流社会名媛和肺病患者也不乏相同之处：苍白、消瘦、虚弱。随着结核导致的死亡越来越常见，它在文化各个领域的地位也越来越重要。在结核病的历史上，对它的浪漫刻画并非主流，时间也很短暂，它给那些受害最深之人——城市贫民——的生活带来的巨大影响盖过了一切。然而那些身患结核的浪漫诗人或是喜欢倚靠在沙发上脸色苍白的女子形象仍深入人心。

19世纪，结核病在文化史上有了更重要的地位，当时最富声名的医生也纷纷研究结核，正是因为它在人群中很常见。它是

19世纪致死率最高的疾病。随着工业发展和巴黎、伦敦等拥挤不堪的大都市的扩张，结核发病率快速增加。1862年，马克思和恩格斯写道："工人所患的结核和其他肺病是资本主义存在的必要条件。"工业化、城市化和结核病如此密不可分，以至于1930年代它们被看作国家通往现代化的必经之路。第二次世界大战之前非洲和印度的结核发病率开始增加时，人们将它称为"文明病"。1930年代晚期，英国结核病专家兼印度结核病况评论员莱尔·卡明斯评价说，如今的印度处于英国"发明珍妮纺纱机的年代"。在东非有着丰富经验的英国医生查尔斯·威尔科克斯在距离马克思和恩格斯一个多世纪后，谈到结核发病率在新兴东非城市的攀升时写道："这样的生活催生了如此恶劣的生活条件，其中毫无对人尊严的关怀，人更像是生产机器而不是独立的个体。"结核成了现代化严酷生存条件的象征——以急剧的城市化、工业化和工人阶级的诞生等为表现的现代化。

发展中国家20世纪的经历正是欧洲国家19世纪所经历过的。虽然很难找到相关的历史记录，不过结核显然是当时致死率最高的疾病。19世纪上半叶，西欧的结核死亡率是3‰～5‰。与此相对，如今美国的结核死亡率是百万分之一。18世纪末到19世纪中期，结核在英国的工人阶级中间大肆流行，造成了大规模的伤亡。英格兰和威尔士的1 800万居民中每年都有5万人死于结核，而在霍乱最严重的年份有4万人因此丧生。

从大约1850年开始，结核发病率开始呈持续一百多年的下降势头，这是不争的事实，不过这并不意味着穷人和工人阶级不再受结核所苦。他们仍然受到结核的威胁，而且占结核病人的

76

77

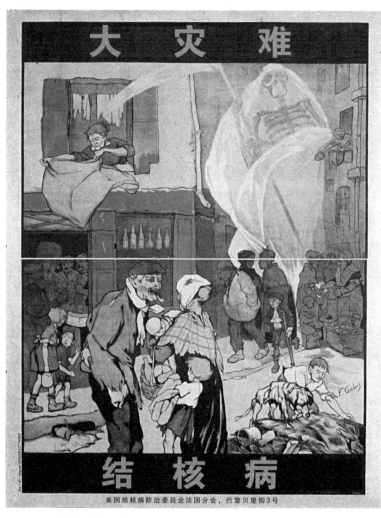

美国结核病防治委员会法国分会，巴黎贝里街3号

图6 欧洲城市的贫民窟生活条件利于结核的传播。这幅1917年的宣传画展示了巴黎贫困街区的景象。死神潜伏在画面的后方

比例非常大。有了可查的历史记录后就证实了人们根据印象做出的判断。1880年代，伦敦儿童医院的尸检表明结核导致的死亡数占总死亡数的45%；80%的死亡儿童来自工人家庭。爱丁

堡的情况也同样如此：皇家儿童医院总死亡人数的39%都是由结核导致的；98%的死亡儿童接受了公共救助。结核对英国的影响实在太大，以至于在结核发病率开始下降之后，英国的总死亡率也随之下降。法国、德国、俄国或美国都有相似的规律：结核发病率随着工业化的推进越来越高。1850年代，在巴尔的摩、费城、新奥尔良和亚特兰大等城市，总死亡人数中的15% ～ 30%由结核导致。和欧洲大部分地区的情况一样，在美国结核也是最主要的死因。与英格兰和威尔士相似，结核发病率在19世纪中期开始下降。不过下降趋势存在差异：不同城市和不同阶级之间下降程度不同；少数族裔患结核病的比例也格外高。

1882年早春，罗伯特·科赫在柏林发表演讲，震惊了整个医学界。他发现了19世纪的头号杀手，他称之为结核杆菌。科赫的发现意义重大，对医学和公共卫生的影响深远。至此结核病有了确切的单一病因。而对细菌的过分关注渐渐削弱了导致结核在特定人群中流行的社会和经济因素的重要性。

结核是由特定病因结核杆菌引起的这一观点没有很快被广泛接受，它也没有终结传染理论支持者和反对者的争论。相信疾病不会在人之间传播的人仍然很多，亚瑟·兰塞姆就是有名的支持者。1887年，他在《流行病学会学报》上撰文提出了一个他认为的土壤传播理论的有力例证。尽管兰塞姆相信有结核杆菌，但他认为结核和霍乱一样，只会发生在特定的地方，它不是人传染给人的。兰塞姆认为结核是臭味引发的："实际上，最有可能的是，为了疾病的有效传播，细菌毒性增加必须发生在体外，这通常是空气中腐烂的动物气味造成的，换句话说是因为通风不足。潮湿泥土的辅助作用也很明显。"不过到20世纪早

78

期,大部分人都相信结核是会传染的。1897年,在卫生委员赫尔曼·比格斯的影响下,纽约将结核列为"传染性疾病",政府施行强制报告制度。有些州会强制病人入院——一些人认为这是为公共利益而侵犯个人自由。

结核杆菌的发现值得庆贺,同时也让人们做出了过分乐观的预测。《伦敦时报》写道:"结核杆菌所引发的疾病每年夺去成千上万条生命,在不远的将来,人们将不再受到这种可怕疾病的侵袭。"媒体对此前景感到欢欣鼓舞。在科赫发现结核杆菌后不到十年,他认为自己已经找到了治疗方法,世界为之沸腾。然而从结核杆菌中提取的结核菌素并没有像科赫所想的那样起到预防作用(不过它是有效的诊断方法)。事实证明发现病因只是解决问题的一部分。

为了防治结核,政府发起了禁止随地吐痰的活动,并且试着修建环境更好的住房。当时最流行的疗法——也是最没有效果的——是到疗养院休养。第一个疗养院建立在西里西亚山区,修建的原因之一是人们相信结核在到达某个海拔后就不会发病。1859年德国出现了最早的疗养院,随后北欧各地都修建了疗养院,20世纪初疗养院的热潮传到了美国。建立疗养院的初衷是让病人暂时远离喧嚣的城市,呼吸乡村的新鲜空气;人们希望病人可以通过休养恢复健康。因为没有积极的治疗方法——当时还没有药物和疫苗——从某种程度上疗养院体现出发现结核杆菌前人们对结核的看法:让病人离开利于结核传播的环境,到没有疾病的地方去生活。

海拔和结核有关的观念后来发生了变化,不过人们仍然相信健康的户外生活对治疗结核有好处。在美国,拉拉森·布朗

79

于1916年出版的《肺结核疗愈指南》和S.阿道弗斯·诺普夫于1899年出版的《作为常见病的结核及其防治》等书中倡导的所谓"户外生活疗法"成为治疗结核的手段。在位于纽约萨拉纳克湖的疗养院里，爱德华·特鲁迪不遗余力地提倡这种疗法，病人不畏冬日的严寒躺在户外，希望清冽的空气能赶走结核。尽管哪怕户外疗法最有力的倡导者也不确定清冽的空气是否真的有助于治疗结核，特鲁迪的疗养院仍受到了极大的欢迎：人们从四面八方到这里来疗养。慈善家赞助穷人疗养；富人自己修建木屋。特鲁迪的疗养院是私人建造的，其他疗养院则是公立的。州政府、市政府都设立了疗养院，联邦政府也为印第安人设立了疗养院。英国和西欧大部分国家的疗养院也都是政府建造的。大部分疗养院都没有萨拉纳克湖周围的田园风光，但都强调休息、健康饮食和进行大量户外活动。

　　人们还尝试了其他办法来治疗结核。休养疗法的本质是被动的，病人主要是休息。外科治疗则大不相同。萎陷疗法或称人工气胸是最常见的肺结核疗法，它通过使肺塌陷、让肺组织松弛从而达到治愈的效果。就像美国结核病专家埃斯蒙德·隆1919年在文章中所写的："人工气胸理论很简单……它跟卧床和整天躺在靠背'治疗椅'上休息是一样的，都是有目的的休息，强制性地让病变部位得到休息。"尽管隆不愿公布"详细数据"，但传闻这种方法对他所说的"严重病例"是有效的。这种疗法对个别病例肯定有疗效，但人工气胸无法解决结核这样一种公共卫生问题，疗养院也同样不能。虽然这些疗法很流行，对一些病例也可能有效，但都无法对公共卫生产生影响。即使有效，这些疗法也只能服务于少数人。

80

从19世纪中期到抗生素问世，因为特定公共卫生措施的实施和生存条件的改善，发达国家特别是美国和英国的结核发病率显著下降。部分出于防治结核的目的，美国一些城市成立了新的卫生部门。不过结核整体发病率的下降不能归功于单一的原因。在英国，人们把工厂里的病人隔离开来，降低了传染的风险，从而降低了人群结核发病率。纽约也是如此：新成立的公共卫生部门帮病人确诊，将他们隔离开来，送到结核病医院救治，避免他们和人群的接触，减少了传染，疗养院也以同样方式发挥了一些作用。减少传染风险自始至终都是控制结核的关键。不过只有在生活条件得到改善的地区才有所需的资源。生活条件无法改善，传染就得不到控制。

结核仍然是穷人才会得的病。在纽约，大量移民聚居在拥挤而缺乏通风的房子里。当地的结核发病率比富裕的区要高得多。1890年，曼哈顿上西区的结核发病率是0.49‰。而在移民聚居的曼哈顿下城，结核发病率高达7.76‰。战争期间美国5岁以下黑人儿童的死亡率是白人儿童的3.74倍。在巴尔的摩等城市的黑人中间，感染率丝毫没有下降，生存条件也毫无改善，而在许多地区的白人中间，两者都已实现。1930年代印第安事务局的患病率调查发现，美国西南部约75%的印第安人感染了结核。20岁以上的皮马人全部感染了结核。在萨斯喀彻温省，印第安人死亡人数的29%由结核导致。在抗生素发明前，美国边缘人群的结核发病率毫无下降趋势。但在1944年，赛尔曼·瓦克斯曼的实验室发现了链霉素，人类由此进入抗生素时代，仿佛奇迹突然降临一般：结核这样一种无可匹敌的疾病遇到了克星。不过在主流人群中间，结核发病率早就开始下降，抗生素只不过消灭了结核的残存势力。

当发达国家主流人群的结核发病率开始下降时,其他地方的发病率却上升了。多地调查——新西兰的毛利人、美洲的印第安人、美国和加拿大还有东非和南非的原住民——表明这些人群结核感染率很高,令人担忧。根据肯尼亚卫生官员的说法,到第二次世界大战时结核已经成为肯尼亚人最主要的死因。尽管很难得到具体数字,但调查工作、对收集卫生数据越来越高的重视还有传闻都表明,亚洲和非洲大部分地区以及美洲土著当中结核发病率出现上升。

在结核发病率为何上升的讨论中,各种种族学说一度占据了上风。落后地区的居民——原住民——对结核来说是处女地;他们具有独特的种族易感性;或者说他们没有被"结核化"。这种理论常常被用来解释南非黑人、美洲印第安人和美国黑人的情况。在印度,种族学说并不流行,不过文明进化理论受到欢迎。1933年,孟买的卫生官员表达了对印度现代化、工业化和城市化的信念,这种信念在当时广为流传:

> 据说在许多西方国家结核已经得到了控制,不再流行……印度现在的疫情在哪个阶段还无法确定。有些人认为疫情还没有到达高峰,印度的疫情还处于早期,人口的结核化程度介于非洲人和高度工业化及城市化的欧洲人之间。这种观点不一定正确,不过印度的疫病的确很猖獗。

种族主义的观点很有说服力,但并不是无懈可击。1930年代末,人们收集了越来越多的证据后,这些观点慢慢瓦解。在坦噶尼喀，英国结核病专家查尔斯·威尔科克斯通过大规模的胸片检查发现，非洲黑人其实一直都对结核有抵抗力；结核钙化灶证明了这一点。（同期在美洲印第安人当中开展的类似研究也得出了同样的结论）。威尔科克斯明白他的发现不仅有"理论意义"，还表明"人们有理由相信治疗会产生效果，改善生活条件和加强教育有助于控制结核，这两者也是公共保健的主要任务"。因为威尔科克斯的研究以及种族观点的普遍改变，第二次世界大战结束时大部分结核病医生都摒弃了种族主义学说。结核是因贫穷而生的疾病。不过尽管种族主义观点已经消失，结核却没有消亡。

第二次世界大战前人们没有采取任何措施来解决边缘人口的结核问题。不过很快几方面的进展联合起来，人类进入了结核抗击史上最卓有成效的时期。世界卫生组织和联合国儿童基金会等战后联合国组织的成立是战后开发所谓"第三世界"思潮的重要组成部分——这一思潮背后有着各种各样的动机，例如冷战期间争相笼络人心、人道主义精神以及与新兴消费和劳动力市场有关的经济利益。加上有效治愈结核的抗生素的发现和卡介苗（以1908年研发疫苗的法国生物学家卡尔梅特和介朗的名字而命名）在印第安人中大规模试用取得的积极成效，解决发展中国家结核病问题的时机终于成熟了。1953年，世卫组织准备开展大规模的卡介苗接种，将其称为"人类历史上针对单一疾病所采取的最大规模的行动"。1950年代，终于可以依靠生物技术消灭结核的观念开始兴起。就像1958年世卫组织在发言中所说的："研发出有效、易于接受、经济可行的公共卫生措施，并以此为基础设计结核防治项目，如今终于成为可能。疫苗和抗

83

生素是防治项目的两个主要部分。"

　　世界范围内数亿人进行了卡介苗接种，抗生素也大有可为。不过结核防治仍面临重重困难。乐观和悲观的情绪相交织——关于卡介苗的疗效出现了互相矛盾的结果，如何保证抗生素在实际中有和试验同样显著的疗效，这些问题深深困扰着人们。验证卡介苗和抗生素的功效成了世卫组织、联合国儿童基金会和英国医学研究委员会的工作重点，在印度和肯尼亚更是如此。疫苗带给人们巨大的希望是因为它可以预防结核，而抗生素可以治疗结核。然而卡介苗的功效差异很大。第二次世界大战前，卡介苗在法国和比利时殖民地得到了广泛应用，相关结果证明了它的预防作用。1946年，对照试验似乎表明卡介苗在美洲印第安人当中效果很好。不过当卡介苗推广到全球时，预防效果却不尽如人意。1979年，人们公布了有史以来规模最大的临床试验结果，卡介苗在南印度的36万名受试者身上毫无效果。疫苗效果的巨大差别始终没有得到合理的解释。人们提出了各种各样的解释——疫苗中的菌株不同、感染过环境中的分枝杆菌、感染率太高、光照影响疫苗效用等等。而在几十年的时间里，人们之所以继续使用卡介苗是因为希望它会有效，另外很重要的是没有其他的预防措施可用。

　　抗生素无疑是有效的。不过在推广使用抗生素的地区中，有些无法进行有效监管；存在药品供应不足的问题；有些药物的配伍价格高昂、有毒副作用或是给药很困难。面对这些挑战，世卫组织和英国医学研究委员会的科学家开发出了更便宜的药物，他们还证明在家服药也是可行的。然而所有的人力、专业知识和取得的突破都无法战胜一个在某些地区很严重，甚至有时是难以克服的问题：耐药性。在不到十年的时间里，肯尼亚从一个没有抗生素的国家变成了1960年代中期耐药性结核几乎泛滥成灾的国家。在其他没有有效的抗生素管控的国家也出现了同样的情况。而在几十年中，世卫组织和其他机构选择对此置之不理，或是弱化问题的严重性。

战后控制结核的努力和同时期的消灭疟疾（以失败告终）及消灭天花（成功实现）运动一起，都是单纯地依靠生物医学来控制疾病。这对抗击结核病来说远远不够。人们对这种方法提出了质疑，比如1950年代印度就爆发了对大规模卡介苗接种的激烈抗议，但这些反对的声音很少得到重视。虽然在印度和其他地方，改善生活条件是降低结核患病率的关键这一观点被人们所接受，但这太不现实，只有持有发展观念的人会这么想。更多人赞同美国结核病专家沃尔什·麦克德莫特的观点，他声称因为生物医学的进步，结核"可以被彻底根除，而**不需要**等到社会基本设施得到改善"。

1970年代中期，人们对全球结核控制的热情已经消退，相关研究也终止了。结核成了被忽略的疾病，但它并没有消失。仍在研究结核的医生和面临感染风险的病人迎来了最艰巨的挑战：艾滋病。

因为艾滋病病毒（HIV）会削弱免疫系统，因此成了结核病的完美搭档。HIV阳性的病人更容易感染结核，HIV也使得潜伏结核感染者很容易转成阳性。1987年两名研究员写道："这两种疾病的结合将来会夺去无数人的生命。"问题的严重程度使得世卫组织和国际结核与肺病防治联合会在1994年警告人们："艾滋病和结核的共同流行将带来本世纪前所未有的公共卫

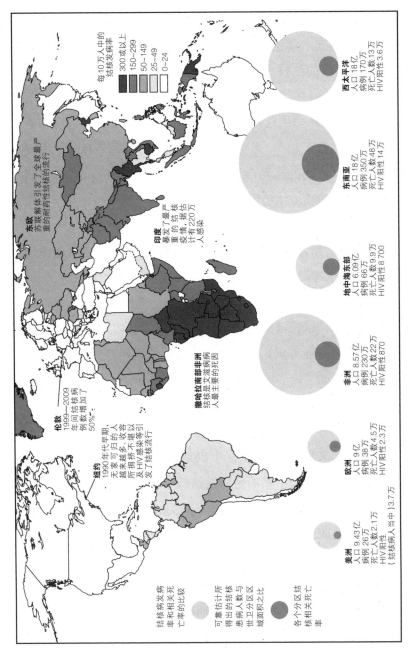

图 7 人们感染结核的风险并不相同，有些地方人们的患病率比其他地方要高

87

生危机。"尽管人们很早就认识到了两种疾病的关联，在艾滋病开始流行的三十年里却没有采取任何措施来遏制事态的发展。2010年，著名的结核和艾滋病专家安东尼·哈里斯和几个同事一起，斥责政府在结核和艾滋病疫情应对上"毫无担当、反应迟缓、缺乏协调。如果这是在战争中……我们的表现会被看作心不在焉和徒劳无功"。撒哈拉南部非洲的疫情最严重。很大程度上由于艾滋病的出现，结核患病率从1990年的1.46‰升高到2003年的3.45‰。结核现在是艾滋病人的主要死因。几十年来一些因素共同造成了结核和艾滋病的蔓延：1970年代末人们对结核的漠视、新发疾病和已有疾病的结合、早期对非洲艾滋病疫情的忽视、全球抗击艾滋病过程中缺乏连贯性和领导等等。

越来越严重的多重耐药性结核使得艾滋病和结核的联合疫情更加棘手。尽管常常被看作新问题，但它其实是1950年代和1960年代肯尼亚等国家出现过的耐药性结核问题的延续，只不过变得更严重了。多重耐药性结核的患者至少是对异烟肼和利福平这两种最常见最有效的抗生素耐药。广泛耐药性结核——对异烟肼或利福平还有至少一种氟喹诺酮和注射药物耐药——表面上看起来是新问题，实际上也是由来已久。多重耐药性和广泛耐药性结核与早期的耐药性结核一样，都是各个层面对抗生素使用不善的结果：病人不服药；感染防控不力；药物短缺；项目管理失职；过去认为耐药性结核不是大问题；现在认为治疗多重耐药性结核不划算，不过这种观念慢慢在改变。就像艾滋病和结核联合一样，多重耐药性结核也被人们忽视了。如今

因结核死亡的人比历史上任何时期都多。

流　感

　　1918年席卷全球的两波流感以及1919年的第三波流感是继鼠疫之后历史上最严重的大流行病。过去也曾经有流感流行——最近也最严重的一次在1889—1892年间，但没有一次能和第一次世界大战期间流感的严重程度相比。这次流感造成至少5 000万人死亡。死亡集中在灾难性的10月和11月。回顾这次疫情，《英国医学杂志》在1919年4月撰文写道，孟买的流感疫情"造成的混乱……只有鼠疫能相提并论"。当时人们还不知道病毒来自何处，而亚洲常常被提及。在意大利，坊间流传这根本不是流感，而是德国人发起的化学战。一名意大利医生制作了题为《最新的严重流行病是否是阴谋？》的宣传册，公然发问。已知最早的疫病于1918年3月5日在美国堪萨斯的芬斯顿营地暴发，随后传播到其他要塞和军事基地。4月病毒出现在开往法国的客船上。接着疫病在欧洲快速传播开来，抵达北非和印度，到7月中国和澳大利亚都出现了疫病。在菲律宾，许多码头工人都感染流感而病倒了，港口陷入了瘫痪。4个月内疫病就播散到了全球。

第二波流感流行比第一次要严重得多，于1918年8月在法
国最先暴发。借助海洋贸易和运兵船，疫病很快播散到了世界
各地，同期出现在了波士顿、法国的布雷斯特和塞拉利昂的弗里
敦，接着顺着穿越西伯利亚的铁路抵达亚洲北部。印度和英国
军队把病毒带到了伊朗，有10%～25%饱受战争和饥饿摧残的
伊朗人民因此丧生。在日本管辖下的西伯利亚海港城市符拉迪
沃斯托克，病毒随着船只抵达日本。疫病首先袭击了非洲西海
岸的弗里敦，报纸写道，整个国家"一片混乱……人们毫无尊严
地死去……墓地位置不够，人们只得将死者埋在沟渠里"。接着
病毒沿着新修的铁路深入非洲腹地，在毫无预警的情况下抵达
加纳。殖民地的一名官员称在北部"洛哈就像个被废弃的村子，
荒无人烟。我听说人们怀疑是不是世界末日到了"。疫病抵达
开普敦之后，很快就随着铁路传播到了北部。因为有着非洲最
繁忙的港口和最完善的内部交通网络，南非的流感传播非常迅
猛。病毒沿着刚果河在蒸汽船上传播，几乎回到了大西洋岸边。
伴随着印度洋地区的贸易，流感传播到了非洲的另一端，9月下
旬最早出现在蒙巴萨。

在几个月内，第二波流感就蔓延到了地球上几乎每个有人
居住的角落。1919年冬天第三次流感暴发，这次流行更为平和，
到来年春天就结束了。整个流感大流行终于过去了。

流感对人口的影响非常惊人，五亿人被感染，这是全球人口
的三分之一。因为上报不完善和诊断不准确，要得出确切的死
亡数字很困难。在印度和撒哈拉南部非洲这些疫情最严重的地
区，人口统计学数据很少，医务人员人手有限，几乎没有保留相

关记录。而在可能遭受了流感沉重打击的中国，直到1930年代政府才开始有相关的统计数据。考虑到流感的凶猛程度，真实的死亡人数肯定比数据显示的要多。这些年来人们一再修正死亡数据。1927年美国医学会发表了埃德温·奥克斯·乔丹题为《流感流行调查》的论文，文中估计全球死亡人数为2 150万。长期以来人们以这一数字为标准，因为相关的研究太少。不过现在历史学家认为埃德温的估计"低得离谱"。历史学家对流感流行越来越感兴趣，在深入研究之后不断上调了死亡数据，有时调整的幅度很大。人们对俄罗斯和中国的疫情了解得仍然很少，不过最新估计是全球有5 000万人因此丧生；有人认为真实数字可能是这一数字的两倍。

　　流感在有些国家甚至是一些国家的某些地区造成的破坏更为严重；不同年龄和性别的病人死亡率也有差别。澳大利亚、新西兰、美洲的土著的死亡率是其他人群的四倍。在阿拉斯加北部偏远的威尔士村庄，流感成为"处女地流行病"：仅有的310名居民中有157人死亡。据估计印度有1 800万人死亡，死亡人数显然是最多的。和其他地方一样，在印度因流感而死亡的也主要是青壮年，其中的原因不明。这一点和以往以及平常每年的流感主要袭击老人和孩子很不一样。在印度，因为照顾病患，妇女感染流感的比例最高。死亡的多是青壮年，又加上妇女死亡比例高，使得印度接下来几年的人口出生率明显下降——1919年人口出生率下降了30%。流感流行导致妇女数量下降，夫妻一方失去自己的伴侣。

　　这次流感传播到了世界上最偏远的角落。在太平洋岛国，流感造成了灾难性后果——岛上的死亡率比其他任何地方都要高。几乎没有一个国家的死亡人数在总人口的5%之下。西萨摩亚的损失最惨烈：几星期内3 800万居民中有22%死亡。如果同样的情形发生在如今的美国，那意味着会有7 000万人死去。尽管通过严格地隔离到访的乘客和阻止邮船靠岸，美国海军管理局基本上把流感阻挡在了美属萨摩亚之外，西萨摩亚却从来没有采取这些措施。结果，新西兰的蒸汽船"泰伦号"的乘客将流感病毒带到了西萨摩亚。这艘船启航的时候当局给它颁发了无疫证明，然而在它从新西兰开往西萨摩亚期间，新西兰的疫情变得严重起来。西萨摩亚和其他停靠的港口没有接到任何警告。岛民看到"泰伦号"上的报纸才获知疫情，有人直到流感暴发才明白过来。尽管西萨摩亚和新西兰一样属于大英帝国的版图，太平洋沿岸的国家对流感也已经很了解，却没有人警告这些岛国这次疫情异常凶猛，非同一般。几天之内西萨摩亚就沦陷了。90%的岛民感染流感，社会、行政和经济生活陷入瘫痪。

人们将病毒的巨大破坏力归咎于岛民的道德缺陷。英国驻汤加的代理写道："酋长们面对村民的苦难冷漠而无动于衷，这是疫情中最让人难过的事情……疫情最严重的时候……找不到一个汤加人来做那些紧急的工作。"这影响了西方国家对汤加的政策："这次事件让我们不得不重新认识汤加人的品格，他们缺乏深沉的感情，无法承担自治的重任。"95%的发病率使得汤加人无法积极应对疫情。而英国评论家却一面颂扬自己的英勇表现，一面责备岛民的迟缓反应。

西萨摩亚的死亡率令人震惊，疫情过后，人们发出了种种拷问——在如今这样一个交通越来越发达、信息飞速传播的世界里，怎么会发生这样的惨剧？ 1919年夏，英国殖民部成立了萨摩亚流行病委员会,调查邻近的美属萨摩亚成功阻击了疫病,而西萨摩亚和其他岛国却不幸沦陷的原因。问题之一是"上述疫病的侵入和播散是否由帝国官员即新西兰政府或所说的西萨摩亚群岛当局玩忽职守所引起的"。

答案是肯定的。委员会发现政府管理混乱使得流感相关的信息传递不顺畅。进一步调查还发现,西萨摩亚的英国管理者对待疫情疏忽大意;医生们认为先进的医疗技术可以抵挡病毒的猛烈进攻。沟通不畅的问题在其他地方也存在。英国殖民部没有通报任何国家;殖民地国家反倒表现得更负责,一旦本国出现流感就及时通知邻国。信息的传播简直是混乱无序。因为流感不是必须申报的疾病,举例来说,只有在塞拉利昂和赞比亚选择通报邻近的尼日利亚,或是人们读到新闻甚至等到流感已经出现时,殖民地国家的人们才知道发生了流感。

这次流感无疑是一场灾难。流感并不是新兴疾病,1918年的大流感也不会是最后一次。自16世纪以来人类经常遭受流行性疾病的侵袭,而流感的历史更久远,它每年都会暴发。十年前的1889—1890年间就有过一轮疫情,而1957年、1968年和2009年流感也都曾流行,将来可能还会有流感。但1918年的大流感和所有的疫情都不一样。

流感是病毒引起的——流感病毒有三种类型,A型流感是最致命的,播散得也最广。它由动物传播给人类,是一种人畜共患病。引发1918年大流感的病毒人类之前从未见过,直到2005年人们才确定它属于H1N1型流感(H代表血细胞凝聚素,N代表神经氨酸苷酶;这两种都是蛋白)。它有几个与众不同的地方:和以往的流感相比,它感染青壮年的概率大大增加,是其他流感和季节性流感病毒的20倍；青壮年和老人感染后症状也严重得多，感染会很快引发重症肺炎。这次流感的死亡率比以往都要高许多。三波流感疫情接踵而至，人们没有喘息的时间，也来不及准备。

人们至今不明白，1918年的大流感为什么会有这些特点，特别是拥有超强毒性。通过研究保存下来的病毒样本——2005年人们至少对1918年秋的流感病毒进行了完整的基因测序——人们发现它是名为H1N1和H2N2家族的四种人流感和猪流感病毒的远祖。1918年它作为一种全新的病毒出现，可能起源于人，后来传染给了猪。不过现在科学家还没有确切证据，人们也不清楚它是何时分化成人流感和猪流感病毒的。现代猪流感和人流感病毒的基因相似性、人流感和猪流感的长期相关性都让研究人员得出结论，猪可能是动物持续性流感和人类季节性流感之间的媒介。

直到1997年情况才有了变化。当年中国香港暴发了名为H5N1的高致病性禽流感，并直接传染给了人类。不过H5N1只通过家禽传染给人，还没有出现确定的人际传播。人们渐渐发现原来鸟类特别是水鸟才是A型流感病毒的主要携带者。禽流感可以直接传染人这一发现颠覆了以往的流感传播模型，并且引起了病毒学家——他们曾怀疑有这种可能——和卫生官员的警惕。流感除了可以直接在动物和人类之间传播外，还可以通过抗原漂移（antigenic drift）快速经常发生变异（这就是为什么每个秋季都需要新的流感疫苗）。基因重配是抗原漂移的一种，即不同毒株混合从而产生新的病毒；1918年、1957年和1968年的情况可能就是如此。将来H5N1也可能会发生重配变得可以

94

人传人，引发病毒在易感人群中的大规模流行。

流感病毒如此变化多端，2010年著名流感病毒学家组成的团体共同写道："尽管人类在许多领域包括人类和动物疫情监控及大范围的病毒基因筛选等方面取得了持续进展，然而我们预测和防控流感的能力并不比五百年前更出色，2009年突如其来的全新H1N1流感病毒证明了这点。"

人类对流感已经有了深刻的了解，然而仍有许多未解之谜。流感病毒的复杂性和它的毒力令人受挫。1918年疫病暴发时现代医学正快速发展，人们对查明病因并找到治疗方法有了信心。不过直到1940年代疫苗问世前，人类对流感都毫无办法。

不过医学界当时不这么想。1890年代，人们误以为流感是一种细菌感染引起的，这种细菌以发现者德国感染病学家约翰·弗里德里希·法伊弗的名字命名，叫法伊弗菌。流感期间涌现出了一大批疫苗和各种各样的疗法，可惜都没有效果，细菌学没有发挥作用。直到病毒学发展成熟，科学家才最终于1933年确定流感是病毒引起的。流感期间没有有效的预防和治疗措施。[95]

殖民地国家的殖民者常常批判传统疗法，想用现代医学取而代之，不过现代医疗技术治疗流感的效果并不比传统疗法明显。殖民地官员和呼吸科医生记录下了人们对现代医学的不满，人们变得越发信赖传统术士。在孟买，人们对阿育吠陀和尤纳尼医学重新燃起兴趣。在塞拉利昂，殖民地当局对疫情的应对引得《塞拉利昂周报》的编辑写道："这次疫情应该成为国家历史标志性的起点。事情已经越来越明白……我们的幸福要靠自己，我们要独立自主。"尽管没有实际有效的方法，医生仍然给出各种建议。在津巴布韦南部的贝林圭，当地官员称将芥泥、蔻麻油、白兰地和"肺炎合剂"混在一起给病人使用,取得了"明显疗效"。还有人用石蜡和糖来治疗。殖民地官员和医生一开始对这些疗法充满信心,后来终于承认非洲人认为这些"疗法"都是"江湖骗术",事实也的确如此。内政部不得不承认,人们"不再相信西医的疗效",医生和诊所在劝说人们放弃传统医术上取得的进展前功尽弃。非洲人认为吃西药会让人生病,甚至死去。在津巴布韦南部有些地区,当地人会保守疫病暴发的消息,害怕病人被送到可怕的隔离医院去,或者被迫吃下他们认为比流感更有害的西药。这并不是说非洲传统医学对治疗流感很有效果,也不是说摒弃西医转向阿育吠陀医学对阻击疫病有帮助。情况不是这样。所有的医学流派都没有任何效果。

南非的布隆方丹刚发生流感时,当局低调应对。他们认为布隆方丹非常安全,在旅游指南中称这里是"南非的疗养地"。当地人相信布隆方丹可以把流感拒之门外,到了10月上旬流感在西非造成大量死亡的时候,当地报纸上的文章还在猜测"常见的普通流感"能有多致命。很快随着死去的人越来越多,医院人满为患,人们这才了解这次疫情的严重性。10月下旬,荷兰归正教会的一名长者说:"我感觉就像世界末日。"在疫病的巨大冲击之下,政府积极行动起来——关闭影院和学校;要求当地医生免费给公众提供"流感冲剂";征召南非黑人为死者挖掘墓穴。

英国拥有最完善的公共医疗设施,对流感的应对却是最无力的。医生对细菌理论充满信心,相信自己能战胜流感,不肯承认没有有效的预防和治疗药物。另外,许多医学人士认为恐慌情绪会促进流感的蔓延,人们在慌乱中会四处传播疾病。因此卫生官员呼吁人们保持冷静。加上对现代医学的迷信,使得政府低估了疫情的真正严重程度。《英国医学杂志》等出版物建议不报道疫情，不采取任何措施；一名编辑写道，"疫病总会造成伤亡。发表这样的报道时更谨慎一些难道不比大肆宣扬造成恐慌好吗？"《曼彻斯特卫报》的编辑也发出了同样的感叹："恐惧会加重疫情，假如能让人们不被恐惧裹挟，攻克疫病一定能取得很大的进展。"政府不愿采取积极的举措，在战时更是如此。12月《泰晤士报》感叹道："自黑死病以来没有一次瘟疫横扫全球；或许从来没有像这样任其发展，听之任之。"

听从了医生的建议，伦敦地方政府除了要求剧院加强通风外，没有采取任何措施。因为对细菌理论深信不疑，错误地相信 97预防和治疗药物即将问世，政府没有调配足够的资源来应对疫情。第一次世界大战极大地影响了疫情——人们对战胜疾病的信心、医生人手（许多都入伍了）、资源等方方面面都受到了影响。让英国人民在国外作战的同时抵抗国内的疫病，被证明是一项艰巨的任务。地方政府委员会的首席医疗官阿瑟·纽肖姆写道：

有时国家会面临这样的情况，人们的主要责任是要"继续工作"，哪怕生命和健康会受到威胁。面对流感情况就是如此……生产军需品的工人和从事有关国家安危工作的人们必须履行这种责任……在上述种种情况当中，如果能将病人隔离，如果在工厂、厂房、兵营和舰船上，能严格地隔离病患、增加人与人之间的距离，如果能不顾一切避免人员密集，或许能够挽救生命、控制感染播散、让人们免于病痛。然而，人们必须"继续工作"。

98

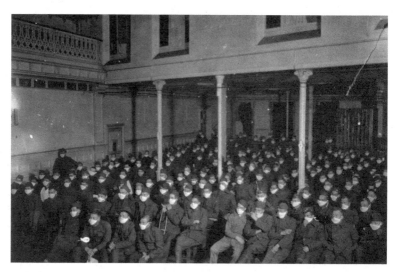

图8　第一次世界大战期间，因为害怕流感，士兵们在法国戴着口罩看电影

　　1918年秋在英格兰，几个星期里流感就夺去了25万人的生命。因为战争而分散了精力的医生和他人没有认真地对待疫病，不过仍然有许多人意识到了事态的严重性。《泰晤士报》写道："灾难如此深重，疫病四处泛滥，人们因为饱受战争恐怖的折磨而拒不接受事实。流感就像飓风席卷过生命的原野，夺走成千上万年轻的生命，留下受病痛所苦的人们，而在我们这一代，这些惨痛的牺牲将得不到认可。"

　　在美国，公共卫生部门一开始在印发的宣传册上声称，现行流感严重程度大体上和季节性流感近似。1918年10月的头几个星期，即使病例数不断增加，纽约市的卫生委员仍然对疫情的严重性轻描淡写。因为相信市政府能控制疫情，他敦促市民们保持冷静，宣称恐慌会使情况更糟糕。在意大利，随着紧张和恐慌情绪的加剧，民事当局要求最有影响力的《意大利晚邮报》停止公布流感死亡人数。这些城市在意识到疫情的严重性后改变了起初的轻慢态度，积极采取措施应对。然而仍然没有出现有效的药物。

尽管在抵御流感的过程中没有发挥有效作用，现代医学的地位仍没有丝毫动摇。实验室变革引领了新时代的到来，而且已经无法回头。不过许多医生和公共卫生专家坦承自己能力有限。回想起1919年的大流感，细菌学家弥尔顿·J.罗西瑙在《美国医学会杂志》上发文称："我们从疫情中学到的唯一东西就是我们对流感一无所知。"许多人都持有同样诚实的态度，这并没有让人们对医学失去信心，起码在美国如此；它促使科学家们找寻新的机遇。

流感大流行的影响无法估量。历史研究大多关注疫情本身而不是它的后续影响。对疫病最感兴趣的是生物医学家而不是历史学家。H5N1型流感和2009年猪流感的暴发——没有达到预期的全球流行的程度——激发了人们对研究1918年大流感起因和后果的极大兴趣。这次流感对20世纪和21世纪的病毒学发展起到了深远的影响。不过还有许多历史问题没有找到答案。有几点是明白无疑的。其中一点是，因为疫病在太平洋岛国造成的灾难，以及新西兰和南非对将流感列为法定报告类疾病的呼吁，人们建立了帝国范围内的疫情监测和报告系统。直到二战前这一系统都没有发挥作用，不过疫病唤起了人们对建立全球流感监测系统的兴趣——监测系统现在要有效得多。

这次大流感对文化、经济、政治、社会和人口等又有哪些影响呢？从我们有限的了解看来，它对美国似乎没有影响。人们几乎已经将它遗忘。人们的记忆和文献记载中找不到它的踪迹。除了少数几本专门研究流感的书，它在这段历史上很少被着重提及。可是在有近2 000万人因此而丧生的印度，情况也是如此吗？或许是的，但我们无法确定。

非洲许多国家——例如津巴布韦、尼日利亚、扎伊尔和南非——涌现出了一批五旬节（或称灵性）教堂。受上帝指引的先知现身人间，要将人们从流感的病痛中拯救出来，教堂因此而成立，尼日利亚的主教堂和扎伊尔的金邦谷教堂都是在这个时期成立的。流感暴发后不久就成立的津巴布韦五旬节教堂，在疫情结束后仍得以长期保留。

在南非的布隆方丹，疫情影响下，政府及时对公共卫生法做出了一系列修改并着手进行济贫工作，他们不得不承认布隆方丹也存在疫情，也有贫民窟。"疫情所曝光的贫民窟和惨状……让人们感到震惊。"镇书记员兼会计说。当地的《友人》报写道："疫情的直接结果是促使公众良知朝着迟来的社会改革的方向发展。过去被认为是不切实际的空想，现在成为亟待解决的事项，计划也被提上了日程。"人们之前也提出过改革方案，而疫情的冲击才让人们真正行动起来。就像市长对流感委员会所说的，"市里早就考虑过相关计划，疫情的到来加快了事情进展，引起了公众关注，改革的时机已经成熟了"。目前我们只能猜测疫情在其他城市也引发了同样的改革，但它对生活其他方面的影响还无法确认。

1918年的大流感是一次事件。与疟疾和结核这些持续存在的大流行病不同，流感暴发了，又慢慢平息下来。从这个意义上说，它更像天花或鼠疫。当然这两者已经不再是威胁全球的疾病了，但流感仍然是。1997年H5N1型流感在人群中暴发，2009

年新型H1N1毒株出现，引起了人们对类似1918年大流感的担心。这些担心还没有变成现实，我们不知道灾难何时会降临。我们就和17世纪的英国人民一样。他们知道潜伏着的鼠疫随时会暴发，对此已经无奈地接受。他们不知道鼠疫会在何时因为何种原因而暴发，不过他们知道它会怎样发动袭击：搭乘船只从境外而来。一旦得知消息，将流行病阻挡在国境外来自保，是阻止流行病暴发的唯一可能方式。现在我们有了疫苗和有力的全球监测系统，一些地区也拥有了运行良好的公共卫生设施。然而我们仍然和17世纪的先辈们一样，紧张不安地等待着流行病的入侵。

另外，一旦致命的疫病暴发，公共卫生设施缺乏、无法获取预防性药物、免疫系统受损和联合感染等导致结核和疟疾在资源匮乏的地区至今仍造成危害的因素，同样将会使得流感大流行如在1918年那样带来广泛影响。

现在我们对战胜流感的困难已经有了充分了解，病毒学家和卫生官员不像1918年大流感时一样过度自信，因此流感很难再唤起人们的关注。对许多人来说，流感和普通感冒没有区别。1976年的猪流感和2009年的H1N1型流感都远远没有达到公共卫生官员所预测的严重程度。这都使得人们对严重疫情的担忧产生了松懈。人们不应该如此。

艾滋病

艾滋病的出现终结了人类的狂妄。当人们以为即将要消灭所有传染病时，艾滋病却以猛烈的势头袭来。明白这一点后，医学可以消灭所有传染病这样的吹嘘消失了，世界上将不再有瘟疫这样的希望也破灭了。

20世纪早期，艾滋病就在中非蔓延开来，直到1981年春，洛杉矶和纽约的医生发现肺孢子菌肺炎（一种真菌感染，免疫功能受损的人容易患病）和卡波西肉瘤（一种罕见癌症，老人多见）这两种罕见病的发病率上升，艾滋病才以现在人们熟知的形式进入公众视野。发病率突然上升本来就很反常，更奇怪的是这些病例都集中在性生活活跃的同性恋男性身上。大约一年之后，血友病患者和注射吸毒者当中也出现了类似疾病。海地也出现了同样的病患。一名关注美国疾控中心新闻的比利时医生彼得·皮奥特发现，美国的情况和他在安特卫普的诊所里的情况有些相似——诊所经常有非洲移民来就诊。世界各地也出现了越来越多关于卡波西肉瘤不明病例和其他免疫系统疾病的报道。这些群体之间有何关联？为什么他们会患上这些罕见而且免疫功能正常的人都不会得的病？这引起了医学界的关注。一开始（很不幸），美国疾控中心把它叫作同性恋相关免疫缺陷症。1982年夏天，科学家将其正式命名为获得性免疫缺陷综合征（AIDS），这一名称沿用至今。不久以后，法国的巴斯德研究所和美国国立癌症研究所分别于1983年和1984年分离出相关病毒。两家机构分别给病毒命名，每家机构都声称自己独立发现了病毒。不过很快医学界就病毒名称达成了一致：它被称为人类免疫缺陷病毒（简称HIV）。

目前在世界范围内已经有近7 500万人感染艾滋病，近3 000万人死亡。每年都有上万起新发感染病例。世界各地都出现了艾滋病病例。不过发病率存在差异：三分之一以上的感染和死亡病例都聚集在南部非洲。在中东、拉丁美洲、日本和欧洲一些地区，感染艾滋病的大部分是边缘群体；而在非洲的中部、东部和南部，艾滋病是普遍疾病。2004年，斯威士兰的产前诊断诊所的数据显示患病率高达42.6%。

艾滋病引起医学界关注两年后，人们就找出了致病的病毒，和其他流行性疾病病原体的发现过程比较起来，这是了不起的进步——发现鼠疫的病因花了上千年的时间。这都要归功于几十年里分子生物学、免疫学和病毒学取得的进展。短时间内就发现了病毒，而美国联邦政府又在医学研究上源源不断地投入（美国在艾滋病研究上的投入比其他国家要多得多），这使得人们草率预言疫苗将很快问世，同时在一段时间里增强了现代医学对自身的信心。

然而乐观情绪没有维持多久。发现病毒还远远不够。HIV

104

是一种复杂的逆转录病毒,有不同的亚型。实际上HIV有两种分型:HIV-1和HIV-2。前者更常见;HIV-2造成的感染主要发生在西非,它更不容易传染,播散速度慢得多。HIV-1分成3个亚型组(M型、N型和O型),并进一步分成11个不同的基因亚型(A到K)。M型是导致流行的主要亚型,99%的病例都属于此型。基因亚型中的A、C和D占所有病例的大约84%。南非、印度和中国的大部分病例都是C亚型感染导致——因此在全球感染亚型中占据很高比例。

HIV-1和HIV-2都是动物源性病毒,每种亚型都是黑猩猩(携带HIV-1)和白枕白眉猴(携带HIV-2)分别传染给人类形成的。HIV在中非的基因多样性最丰富。中非发现了所有M亚型的HIV,还有许多基因组成发生改变的重组病毒。这种基因多样性表明HIV在中非存在的时间最长,因此中非是疫情的发源地。20世纪初的某个时间,感染了HIV的黑猩猩的血很可能通过伤口或破损皮肤进入猎人体内,把病毒传染给了人类。大约在1920年,病毒传播到了利奥波德维尔(1966年改名叫金沙萨),随后借助不断发展的交通网络传遍了整个非洲。历史上有些时期,有些地方艾滋病传播得特别快:殖民时代人们发起了消灭昏睡病、雅司病和梅毒的运动,治疗过程中经常重复使用针头,从而导致短期内许多人感染。1950年代和1960年代,治疗梅毒时使用未经消毒的针头造成妓女感染,这尤其使得艾滋病病毒进入一般人群之中。大量妓女感染之后,艾滋病很快就播散开来,特别是1960年代利奥波德维尔正经历着社会剧变:人们大规模移居到城市里,失业率高,从事卖淫的人口激增。联合国教科文组织等机构雇用的许多海地人经常在海地和扎伊尔之间往返，艾滋病随之传播到了海地。世界各地随后也都出现了艾滋病。

　　HIV很难控治。首先，它是一种慢病毒，潜伏期很长，病情进展缓慢。包括大部分病毒在内的生物的遗传物质都是脱氧核糖核酸（DNA）。然而HIV是逆转录病毒，它的遗传物质在核糖核酸（RNA）内。HIV侵入宿主细胞后，在逆转录酶的作用下RNA会转变成DNA，插入宿主的DNA当中，随宿主DNA复制扩增。转变的过程中，病毒的复制会出错，导致病毒发生突变。因为HIV变异很快，无法预测，因此研发疫苗非常困难——目前看来是不可能的。HIV通过感染的体液进入体内——主要是血液和精液。异性传播是最常见的。不过，母婴传播、静脉注射时使用未消毒的针头、男性同性恋性行为都是重要的传播途径。HIV进入人体后会攻击免疫系统中的CD4细胞。关键在于它会攻击两种重要的CD4免疫细胞：辅助性T细胞和巨噬细胞，前者是人体抵御异物和感染的主要细胞，后者可以吞噬异物，以便免疫系统识别。感染后会发生血清转化——机体生成HIV抗体并且识别病毒的过程。人们用病毒载量来衡量感染的严重程度，感染早期患者的传染性最强。

　　根据CD4细胞计数可以将感染分成四个阶段，健康人体内每立方毫米血液中CD4细胞的数量大于1 000。第一阶段CD4的数量一般超过500，感染者没有任何症状。第二阶段CD4计数会减少到350～499之间，可能出现体重下降和真菌感染等症状。第三阶段CD4降到350以下，病人的免疫功能严重受损，容易发生机会性感染。病情全面暴发时CD4不足200，即第四阶段。HIV惊人的复杂性和攻击免疫系统的能力是它的主要特征。

106

决定艾滋病防控成效的政治和社会因素使得问题更加复杂。性行为、性别、贫穷、药物获得难易程度以及有无控制疫情的政治意愿都包含在内。艾滋病暴发之际医学取得了巨大成就，那时医学界坚信药物是最好的解决办法并且药物会很快问世，因此在疫情防控上社会和医学层面始终存在着矛盾。广义上说，生物医学界无异取得了突破性成果，由此创造了一个全新的科学产业。短期内人们不断加深了对发病机制的理解。在不到十年时间里，艾滋病就从一种几乎无药可医的绝症变成了可控的慢性病。

然而现实中抗击艾滋病取得的进展和实验室的成就并不一致。尽管已经有了治疗艾滋病的药物，但不是所有人都有药可用，不断出现的新病例也说明预防工作只取得了部分成效。一开始抗击疫病的工作就遇到了无数困难。在美国，艾滋病主要是和性活跃的同性恋男性及注射吸毒者紧密联系在一起的，病人常常会产生慌乱和恐惧情绪，受到道德谴责。保守派参议员杰西·赫尔姆斯等公开指责男同性恋，声称艾滋病是老天对他们的惩罚。政府发起的换针管计划引发了持续的争议，许多人认为这会助长吸毒，事实证明该计划效果显著。许多人认为食品与药品监督管理局等政府机构在新药审批上反应迟缓，效率低下。作为抗议，人们发起了声势浩大的抗击艾滋病的活动，"行动起来"（ACT UP）组织就是一个例子。

倡导安全性行为的活动遭到了禁欲支持者的反对，他们认为禁欲才是预防艾滋病的最好方法；安全套花了很长时间才被狎妓者接受，还有一些人直接拒绝；疫病在美国稳定下来后，安全套的使用率又开始下降。除美国外其他国家应对艾滋病的方式也都大相径庭，无法加以概括。有些国家很被动，有些国家积极采取措施。古巴把所有HIV阳性的患者都严格隔离起来，并且强制要求全民接受HIV检测。在非洲，乌干达从疫病暴发开始就直面病毒，提倡并且鼓励人们洁身自好，减少性伴侣数量。而津巴布韦等国家直接否认境内存在艾滋病患者。

如果从科研投入、发表论文的数量、从业人数和取得的突破等方面来衡量，医学界在抗击艾滋病上的投入是巨大的。政治和社会层面就要逊色一些。2008年，从初期就开始关注疫情的几位著名医生在《柳叶刀》上发表文章称，全球抗击艾滋病时"反应迟缓，重视程度严重不够，行动缺乏统一性和持久性"。

非洲是艾滋病的发源地和疫情中心，这里的疫情却被大大忽视了。其中的原因很复杂，既有内部原因也有外在原因。许多人都认为艾滋病是同性恋才会得的疾病，因此得病被认为是可耻的。乌干达和塞内加尔这两个国家是例外，两国都公开抗击艾滋病，坦承疫情，通过去污名化来努力控制疫情。在南非，时任总统塔博·姆贝基和卫生部长认同美国否定派彼得·迪斯贝格的说法，声称HIV不会引发艾滋病，新开发的药物毫无用处。在这种情况下，1990年代中期否定艾滋病的声音达到了顶峰。

世卫组织迟迟没有做出反应。艾滋病流行四年后，世卫组织总干事哈夫丹·马勒仍然没有将抗击艾滋病作为头等大事。他在讲话中说："艾滋病并没有像野火一样在非洲蔓延开来。每天夺去几百万孩童生命的是疟疾和其他疾病。"另外，非洲的疫情有其独特之处。绝大部分和艾滋病有关的研究都是在美国和欧洲多数地区开展的，而美国和欧洲感染艾滋病的大都是同性恋男性和注射吸毒者。医学研究和政策主要关注的是研究开展国家的艾滋病的特点。起初人们认为异性间的感染很罕见，也不是主要的传播方式。在美国，人们意识到感染艾滋病的主要是"高危人群"后，就放松了警惕；人们所担心的异性性行为传播所导致的艾滋病大暴发也没有发生。

这给非洲带来了巨大的影响。因为在美国异性性行为传播被认为不重要，非洲因异性性行为传播而暴发的艾滋病疫情（刚果SIDA项目的开创性工作对此有详尽的记录）一开始没有得到重视。这也意味着妇女感染艾滋病的风险没有引起注意。等到1987年世卫组织启动抗击艾滋病的专门项目（后来被重命名为"全球抗击艾滋病项目"，简称GPA）时，疫病已经悄无声息地传播开来了。

随着GPA项目启动和乔纳森·曼（他是刚果SIDA项目的负责人，后来成了抗击艾滋病的传奇人物）受聘成为项目主管，艾滋病在世界范围内得到了前所未有的关注，世卫组织收到的捐赠暴涨。GPA在和乌干达及泰国共同合作减少病毒传播的工作中取得了显著成效，曼也成功取得了非政府组织的帮助。为了减少污名化，确保感染者不受歧视和迫害，GPA把艾滋病变成了一个人权议题。世卫组织在了解到艾滋病曾经并且将继续显著影响结核的发病率后，一度打算联合抗击结核和艾滋病。GPA项目很大程度上是自治的——这在一定程度上导致了项目的最终失败，GPA也是世卫组织规模最大、资金最充足的项目。1987年秋，马勒和曼在联合国大会上发言，这是历史上疾病首次被提上大会的议事日程。世卫组织领导了全球抗击艾滋病的运动。

109

然而艾滋病受到广泛关注的时间并不长。在和时任世卫组织总干事的中岛宏反复发生摩擦后，乔纳森·曼于1990年提交了辞呈。GPA项目进展变得缓慢起来。不久之后，世卫组织就终止了该项目。抗击艾滋病的工作交由联合国艾滋病联合规划署（UNAIDS）来承担，旨在巩固某个国家或地区艾滋病工作所取得的成就。从曼的任期结束到联合国艾滋病联合规划署真正开始运作这段过渡时间里，全球抗击艾滋病的工作缺乏领导，处于混乱状态。

不过真正关注全球艾滋病的人本来就不多。因为忙着应付国内的疫情，美国民间抗击艾滋病运动和美国政府基本上对发展中国家的疫情不闻不问。不幸的是，正是在这段时间里非洲的感染人数呈指数增长。GPA项目早期艾滋病受到了全球瞩目，然而人们的热情很快消退了。到1990年代早期，尽管大部分感染者都在发展中国家，但投入到那里的资金只占全球预防艾滋病资金的6%。因为长期以来对疫情的忽视和小心翼翼的政治考量，1990年代人们失去了对抗疫情的宝贵时机。联合国艾滋病联合规划署在发布的全球应对疫情的长篇报告中坦承：出现首例艾滋病病人后的15年内，"社会各部门的领导者面对新挑战表现出的漠视令人震惊"。

除了对疫情的忽视，从1980年代开始直到1990年代，对发展中国家的总体援助也大大减少。里根当政时的美国等捐助国拒绝缴纳会费，世卫组织等联合国机构深受影响（不过GPA项目曾经是个例外，它有专项基金）。新自由主义经济政策导致国家为了偿还大额债务，必须紧缩开支。在最急需资源的时候，结构调整计划占用了国家本就匮乏的资金储备，而艾滋病对经济

110

的巨大影响恰好在此时开始显现。两者叠加的作用非常惊人。其中之一就是医疗保健资金大幅减少；许多非洲国家都开始对医疗服务收取使用费——只有很少的病人才负担得起。

　　同期世卫组织的影响力开始下降，而世界银行的影响力有所增加。从1987年开始，和GPA项目启动同年，世界银行开始资助越来越多的医疗保健项目。这些项目以新自由主义为原则，这意味着人们会以成本效益分析为基础来评估医疗项目；同时也意味着许多国家的公共卫生开支将大幅减少。随着世界银行在资助医疗项目上发挥的作用越来越大，它自然也对项目如何操作有了更大的话语权。其中最有力的影响是从成本效益角度来分析公共卫生措施。1993年世界银行发表了《世界发展报告：卫生领域投资》，在报告中首次提出了这种给项目排序的方法，按照《柳叶刀》杂志编辑的说法，这意味着向全世界表示"全球卫生事务的领袖从世卫组织变成了世界银行"。世界银行试图找出对经济破坏最大——以伤残调整生命年来衡量——治疗起来也相对便宜的疾病。按照这种计算方法，治疗艾滋病无论如何都称不上划算。新问世的抗逆转录病毒药物售价高昂，对低收入国家来说并不合算。而安全套等经济实惠的预防方法却很难被人们接受。

　　如此一来，发展中国家就处在了一个有些尴尬也有些讽刺的境地：发达国家寻求的疗法即高效抗逆转录病毒疗法即将问世，结果发展中国家却被告知药品太贵，他们用不起。想办法预防艾滋病的传播更经济。追求成本效益这一思路促使美国忽视了社会干预措施，一心研发艾滋病药物，而同样的考虑却使得那些最需要药物的人们无法获取研发出的高效药物。

1990年代人们对艾滋病没有足够的重视，失去了阻止疾病蔓延的机会。全球应对艾滋病不力。不过同期生物医学界取得了巨大的突破。1995年和1996年人们研发出了两种抗逆转录病毒药物，这两种药物都通过了临床试验并投入使用：第一种是蛋白酶抑制剂——沙奎那韦；后来又研发出第一代非核苷类逆转录酶抑制剂奈韦拉平。在于温哥华召开的第十一届国际艾滋病大会上，科学家宣布采用由这两类药物组成的三联疗法可以有效抑制艾滋病病毒，恢复病人的免疫功能。

艾滋病不再是一种绝症。奈韦拉平不仅可以治疗HIV感染，还可以防止母婴传播。阻断母婴传播一直是防治艾滋病的难题，而在分娩前给产妇一定剂量的奈韦拉平、婴儿娩出后也马上服用奈韦拉平可以有效阻断母婴传播。在大量应用奈韦拉平的地区，母婴传播感染率大幅下降。不幸的是，直到2002年宪法法院介入前，南非的产前诊所都无法使用奈韦拉平——因为南非总统塔博·姆贝基坚信HIV并不会引发艾滋病。

新药的问世使得艾滋病有望成为一种可控的慢性病，从而改变疫情的走向。可惜这些药太贵了——大多数人都承担不起。这些药每年要花1万～1.5万美元，而且必须终身服用。保证病人用得起药成了重点。与此同时，1990年代后期美国国内和艾滋病相关的死亡率开始下降——仅在1996—1997年间，死亡率就下降了46%。美国国内的疫情渐渐缓和下来，而全球疫情却仍然被忽视。

有些全球卫生事务的领导者声称，治疗发展中国家的艾滋病病人既不经济也不可行，因为这些国家缺乏必要的基础设施。《柳叶刀》上有两篇文章就表明了这种观点。其中一篇文章声称

"撒哈拉南部非洲关于艾滋病预防措施和高效逆转录病毒疗法成本效益的数据表明，预防措施的效益起码是抗病毒疗法的28倍"。另外一篇写道："最具成本效益的是预防艾滋病和治疗结核，而成人的抗病毒疗法以及卫生机构提供的家庭护理是成本效益最低的。"治疗和预防措施两者被对立起来。而人们认为这样严峻的选择是必要的。此外美国国际开发署的署长在对众议院的陈词中说，就算给非洲人提供药物他们也不会正确服用，原因之一是他们不戴手表；非洲人对时间的认知不同，无法严格按时间来服药。

后来情况发生了根本性的转变。从新世纪之初开始，人们看待艾滋病疫情的方式发生了变化。全球卫生成为美国政府和比尔及梅琳达·盖茨基金会等主要慈善组织的关注重点。例如，2000年美国只给全球几百人提供了抗逆转录病毒治疗；2009年9月美国国务院称美国正为250万人提供治疗。

美国增加对艾滋病的资助和改变关注点的原因是什么？答案是药品政策和成本。整个1990年代，治疗耐药性结核和抗逆转录病毒的药品都贵得惊人。全球卫生部门的官员认为这是固定成本而不是人为定价导致的。1980年代早期，"行动起来"这一组织发起了旨在让人们有药可用的抗艾滋病运动。1990年代末期南非涌现出了新一代抗击艾滋病的活动分子，他们要求政府提供抗逆转录病毒药物，回答一些无法回避的问题：政府说药品成本太高是什么意思？这是由谁决定的？谁定的价？在他们看来，如果高价是人为制定的，那人们自然也可以把价格降下来。一旦药品价格下跌，药物治疗不经济这样的说法也就不成立了。

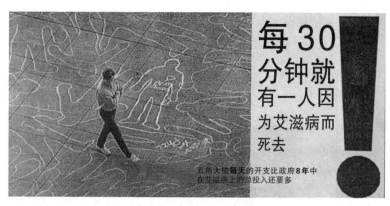

每**30**
分钟就
有一人因
为艾滋病而
死去

！

五角大楼**每天**的开支比政府**8年**中
在艾滋病上的总投入还要多

图9　1980年代和1990年代"行动起来"这一组织让人们开始关注美国政府应对艾滋病的表现，许多人认为政府的反应很迟缓

　　抗击艾滋病的多个领域都开始取得进展。新的研究驳斥了病人服药依从性差以及预防和治疗两者互不相容这些说法。2001年，分别来自海地和开普敦城外卡耶利察的两项关于高效抗逆转录病毒疗法有限效用的研究表明，病人会持续接受治疗。科学家从开普敦研究中更进一步发现：治疗机会增加以后，主动接受检测的人也会增多。也就是说，发现有可靠的治疗方法后，越来越多的人愿意去寻求艾滋病相关的医疗服务。越来越多的人确定了自己是否感染，同时更多的人得到了治疗，因此艾滋病的播散也开始减少。

　　显然在资源匮乏地区，高效抗逆转录病毒疗法也是有效的，但药物的花费仍旧惊人。印度和巴西的制药厂开始生产更廉价的商用抗逆转录病毒仿制药，而其他国家因为专利保护无法生产仿制药。在美国政府和世界贸易组织的协助下，制药企业也努力阻止仿制药品进入全球市场。1997年南非通过了《医药法案》，试图打破这种局面，法案规定，面对艾滋病等公共卫生紧急情况时,国家有权生产和进口仍受专利保护药物的仿制品。

　　1998年,39家制药企业声称该法律侵犯了知识产权,因而向南非的法庭提起了诉讼。抗击艾滋病的活动人士特别是来自"治疗行动"的活动人士反驳道,药品价格与研发过程中的投入严重不成比例,更不必说从人道主义角度考虑应该为人们提供这些药物了。

　　克林顿当局对制药企业的诉求表示支持,他们甚至把南非列入了观察名单——这是施行制裁的前兆,政府声称《医药法案》有"废止专利保护"的可能。副总统戈尔宣布自己将参选总统时,抗议者突然出现在他身后,手中高举着横幅,上面写着:"贪婪害人性命!给非洲提供药品!"其他各地也爆发了抗议,三个月后美国政府就改变了态度:美国政府不会强迫任何国家

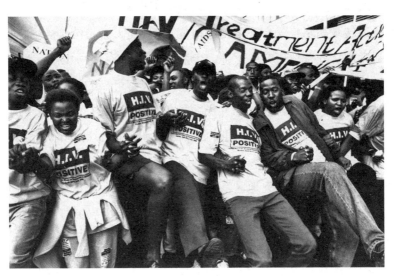

图10　2000年7月,"治疗行动"的示威者在南非德班街头呼吁政府免费提供治疗艾滋病的药品。照片中身患艾滋病示威者的有力形象颠覆了人们对艾滋病的认知和对无助的"非洲"艾滋病患者的成见

购买正品药物,且将会允许仿制药进口。到2001年4月,39家药厂都撤回了诉讼。这样一来,用仿制药来进行治疗的障碍被扫除了。

政府改变药品政策的同时,也大幅增加了艾滋病的资金投入。2003年1月28日,布什总统在发表国情咨文时宣布将制订总统防治艾滋病紧急救援计划(President's Emergency Plan for AIDS Relief,简称PEPFAR),这一举动出人意料,而该计划成为抗击艾滋病的主要资助来源之一。布什总统在讲话中说:

> 艾滋病是可以预防的。抗逆转录病毒药物能够大幅延长病人的生命……能给为数众多的患者提供他们所需要的帮助,这样的机会千载难逢……为了应对境外严重的公共卫生危机,今晚我宣布将设立艾滋病紧急救援计划,这是一项举各国之力援助非洲人民的慈善事业……我敦促国会在未来五年内提供150亿美元资金,其中包括100亿美元新投资金,来遏制受影响最严重的非洲国家和加勒比海地区的艾滋病疫情。

PEPFAR旨在尽快让更多的人有药可用,它在部分程度上仿效了乌干达抗击艾滋病工作的模式。

到2005年抗击艾滋病的资金越来越充足,接受治疗的人数也大大增加,这要归功于下列因素的共同作用:药品价格降低、越来越多的证据表明在资源匮乏地区药物治疗效果也很好、民间抗击艾滋病运动以及PEPFAR等新的资金来源。然而人们获得药物的机会并不均等,同时新发病例表明要阻止艾滋病传播必须进一步增加药品的供给。资金来源也不稳定。污名化和缺乏了解也阻碍着抗击艾滋病工作的进展。哪怕在美国，抗击艾滋病的民间活动非常活跃，拿药也最容易，华盛顿等地非裔美国人的感染率也远远高于白人——2013年的新发病例中有75%是黑人；同样，HIV感染者中也有75%是黑人。2015年印第安纳农村地区注射吸毒者中暴发了艾滋病疫情，有些吸毒者拒绝接受HIV检测，他们担心要是被人看到在当地诊所进出的话会被认为是同性恋，这也反映出耻辱感仍然是大问题；许多人都不知道已经有了治疗艾滋病的药，或是不了解共用针头的危害。

艾滋病从根本上改变了全球卫生状况：为了应对疫情，人们发起了积极而至关重要的民间运动，从而改变了药品定价的规则和人们获取药物的方式，疫情也强化了健康和人权两者的联系。它让我们认识到疾病永远不会从地球上消失。它也提醒我们这是一个机会和资源严重不均等的世界——绝大多数艾滋病患者都生活在发展中国家清楚地揭示了这一点。和其他流行性疾病一样，受艾滋病影响最大的是那些最没有抵抗能力的人们。

117

118

后 记

　　我们要怎样看待人类和大流行病抗争的历史呢？所有过往经历和历史是不是都会对当今有所启发？答案既是肯定的也是否定的。2015年春，世卫组织发表声明，坦承在面对埃博拉疫情时反应迟缓，呼吁大家"吸取教训"。这份声明令人震惊。要等到2015年世卫组织才知道要注重"群体和当地文化"，要埃博拉疫情暴发人们才能发现当地人和其经验的价值，这一切都令人难以置信。世卫组织还说"明白了抗疫能力的重要性"——意思是世卫组织意识到人们没有应对流行病的能力。世卫组织发现"以市场为导向的卫生系统不会投入资源去治疗那些被忽视的疾病"。为何要在埃博拉疫情之后人们才重新意识到如此重要的常识？世卫组织还明白了如果"医疗卫生系统非常脆弱"，人们在疟疾防控或提高产妇存活率等方面取得的进展也会前功尽弃。在2015年之前，人们真的没有吸取这些教训吗？

　　我无意控诉世卫组织——这种情况下它很容易成为攻击的目标——作为全球卫生系统的领导者它能坦承错误是很可贵

的。但无论如何，世卫组织代表了全球卫生领域的人们看待事物的方式。看了世卫组织关于吸取教训的声明，我想强调：世卫组织所吸取的每一条教训（其中有一条教训曾经出现过）在历史上都能找得到。这些经验教训毫无新意：在抗击流行病的历史中，我们一再犯下同样的错误，一再吸取同样的教训。人们缺乏历史意识，这让我感到挫败，不仅仅因为我是一名历史学家，也因为这样既浪费又低效。无视历史同样是幼稚和自大的，这两者的结合会带来致命的后果。以为简单地吸取了教训将来就会不一样是幼稚的，以为能认错就是终于悔过的有识之士是自大的。世卫组织和其他机构必须要问：错误的根源在哪里？比错误本身更重要的是人们为何会犯错。

大流行病不会消亡，未来无疑会出现更多的流行病。它可能来源于流感等人们熟知的病毒，也可能会由新的病毒引发——或许是动物传染给人类的动物传染病。将来我们会怎样应对疫情？既往的模式很可能会重演。那么气候变暖等新的挑战又会怎样影响将来的疫情和人们的应对能力呢？未来随着气候变暖，带病的蚊子很可能会迁徙到新的栖息地。以寨卡病毒为例，2016 年初，由于极端高温形成了适合埃及伊蚊（*Aedes aegypti*，通常被称为黄热病蚊）生存的环境，它所携带的寨卡病毒在拉丁美洲和加勒比海地区大规模暴发。随着其他地区的气温升高，寨卡病毒很有可能会在纬度更高的地方传播开来，而升高的水温可能会有利于霍乱弧菌的繁殖。现在越来越多的证据证明，中世纪晚期的欧洲鼠疫与中亚地区周期性的气温升高有关，我们应该更加关注表明疾病和气候变化有关的其他历史案例。

未来无国界医生等非政府组织会成为可靠的抗击疫情的先锋吗？当整个世界都在观望的时候，是他们勇敢而不知疲倦地 120 战斗在抗击埃博拉疫情的第一线。抑或世卫组织能够重获部分声望？有一点很明确：在严重的大流行病面前，大部分发展中国家的医疗卫生系统都会陷入瘫痪。因此在所有有需要的国家建立强有力的公共卫生系统，是减轻将来疫情可能导致灾难的最有效方式。规模性流行病和大流行病对那些无力应对的国家的影响是最大的，将来也仍然如此。这听起来似乎是常识，然而从世卫组织自埃博拉疫情当中"吸取的教训"来看，人们仍习惯性地将之遗忘。 121

后
记

索 引

（条目后的数字为原文页码，
见本书边码）

索引

D

E

大流行病

大流行病

大流行病

Christian W. McMillen

PANDEMICS

A Very Short Introduction

For Olin, Maya, and Stephanie

Contents

List of illustrations

i

Acknowledgments

Several years ago Nancy Toff at Oxford and I met and discussed a variety of potential projects. I was then in the thick of working on a book on tuberculosis. Writing that book got me interested in epidemics more broadly. Nancy discovered, much to our mutual surprise, that there was no Very Short Introduction on either epidemics or pandemics. Maybe I could write such a book? With Nancy's help I did. Thanks, Nancy. Elda Granata at Oxford has been unflagging in her willingness to answer innumerable questions. She has made the process a pleasure. I am grateful to the students in my course Epidemics, Pandemics, and History for allowing me, without them knowing it, to test this material out on them. This book is based on the hard work of the many historians dedicated to making disease central to human history. My thanks to them. Finally, my wife, Stephanie, and our children, Maya and Olin, deserve, as always, my greatest thanks.

Introduction

This book will introduce readers to the rich history of pandemic and epidemic disease and suggest that much of the way we confront such things now has been shaped by the past. This is an unremarkable statement but an important point. For very often history is forgotten or rediscovered only when we confront contemporary epidemics and pandemics, and thus patterns from the past are repeated thoughtlessly.

What are pandemics and epidemics? An epidemic is generally considered to be an unexpected, widespread rise in disease incidence at a given time. A pandemic is best thought of as a very large epidemic. Ebola in 2014 was by any measure an epidemic—perhaps even a pandemic. The influenza that killed fifty million people around the world in 1918 was a pandemic.

A common way to think about epidemics and pandemics is as events. They come and they go. But if we think about them this way, can we call HIV/AIDS a pandemic? Or tuberculosis? What about malaria? Pandemics can be either discrete events or what I would like to call persistent pandemics. Tuberculosis, malaria, and HIV/AIDS, which affect enormous swaths of the globe and kill millions and millions each year, are persistent pandemics.

In the wake of the 2009 H1N1 influenza pandemic, controversy emerged over the definition of pandemics used by the World Health Organization (WHO) and others. In response, several infectious disease specialists at the National Institute of Allergy and Infectious Diseases at the National Institutes of Health (NIH) came up with a broad framework that can work to help define what a pandemic is and has been. They suggested that it must meet eight criteria: wide geographic extension, disease movement, high attack rates and explosiveness, minimal population immunity, novelty, infectiousness, contagiousness, and severity. It might seem that TB, HIV/AIDS, and malaria are not novel. But their profiles change—TB gets worse in one area, then better in another; XDR-TB emerges—and they become novel again. Each particular historical context is novel. Malaria took on a new identity in the 1950s when the WHO attempted to eradicate it; it took on another in the 1970s and 1980s as the World Bank became the major player in global health. Likewise with HIV/AIDS; its identity has changed so much over time that it has taken on multiple novel identities, each one historically contingent: a death sentence, a chronic and manageable infection, a gay disease, a heterosexual disease.

There are a number of themes and topics that link the history of epidemics and pandemics. The identities of each disease underwent significant change as a result of the late-nineteenth-century laboratory revolution—a revolution that ushered in the age of modern medicine in which we now live. What began with Louis Pasteur in France and culminated with the work of Robert Koch in Germany meant that diseases once explained in myriad ways were forever thereafter explained by one. The consequences of this change cannot be overstated. The discovery of bacteria as the cause of diseases such as tuberculosis meant that centuries-old explanations for disease etiology vanished. For the first time medical science actually knew what caused a given disease. Diseases might actually be able to be cured. The discovery of the tubercle bacillus and the bacteria that caused plague allowed medicine to develop effective therapies, as well as understand how to prevent infections. But the laboratory revolution also cultivated an undue amount of confidence in the power of biomedicine to rid the world of infectious diseases and fostered the belief that the way to do so was far more dependent on attacking germs than on attacking the social conditions that gave rise to disease in the first place.

This points to another pair of themes: the relationship between poverty and disease and the geography of epidemics and pandemics. All of the diseases discussed in this book, while able to be controlled (to varying degrees) by modern medicine, are affected by social conditions. That is, there is a reason cholera disappeared from the United States more than a century ago but is still present in much of the developing world, or that HIV/AIDS disproportionately effects sub-Saharan Africa, or that plague was worse among the poor than the rich during Marseilles's 1720 epidemic. Some places have been able to transcend the conditions that allow infectious diseases to flourish, while others have not.

These days most places with persistent pandemics are in what has come to be called the global south. The burden of epidemic disease has shifted: tuberculosis, once Europe's leading cause of death, has not disappeared from the earth; it has simply moved. TB declined in the West long before any effective therapy or preventive agent existed; it did so because of public health interventions such as isolation and a generally improved quality of life. TB has increased dramatically in the developing world even after the discovery of antibiotics—one of modern biomedicine's triumphs—that actually kill it and cure the patient. It has done so because of conditions that allow it to thrive: unequal access to drugs, crowded living conditions, high rates of infection, and comorbidities like HIV/AIDS, among other things. TB declined in one part of the world without the aid of biomedical interventions and increased in another part of the planet despite them.

None of this means that drugs and medical research are not essential for the control of epidemics. They are, of course.

Antiretroviral therapy, an extraordinary discovery by any measure, has been essential in the fight against HIV/AIDS. Yet access has been uneven, and infection rates are rising in some countries. Since its discovery in the 1960s, oral rehydration therapy for cholera has been lifesaving. But it does nothing to address the reasons why millions of people in the global south are drinking water contaminated by human feces. The very simple point is that there is a relationship between disease and social conditions, conditions that do not exist everywhere and that will not be alleviated with biomedicine.

Fear and dread characterize epidemics. Cholera caused considerable panic in the nineteenth century; those with HIV/AIDS inspired fear and discrimination in places like the United States in the recent past—and into the present. There is still considerable stigma attached to the disease. Plague prompted anti-Jewish pogroms in the fourteenth century. In our own time, the climate of fear in the United States during the 2014 Ebola pandemic was out of proportion to the actual risk. Yet influenza, which has the capacity to kill untold numbers (the 1918 pandemic killed at least fifty million people in less than a year), seems rarely to occasion much concern. Fearing some diseases and not others is often wrapped up in how a given disease manifests—cholera is a thoroughly unpleasant disease, the symptoms of which are dramatic and, to most sensibilities, disgusting—or how it is caused: HIV is tangled up in the complexities of human sexuality; many have perceived its causes to be rooted in social deviance, including intravenous drug use. A disease's place of origin can have an effect on whether it is feared or not. Malaria is now firmly a tropical disease in the developing world. When it appears occasionally in the developed north, it arrives as a frightening and exotic invader.

The question of susceptibility—who gets a disease and why—is important. In early America, colonists considered Indians to be virgin soil for smallpox and other Old World diseases. In the early

4

decades of the twentieth century, black South Africans and others were thought to be racially susceptible to TB, while whites could fight infection. That Africans were less susceptible to malaria than colonists led, in part, to their importation as slaves to the New World in the seventeenth and eighteenth centuries. For hundreds of years, until the bacteriological revolution, many debated whether or not diseases were contagious or brought on by miasma—the bad air caused by rotting animal and vegetable matter. The plague was often considered to be a punishment for sin. Each of these explanations changed.

All of these diseases, save smallpox, are still with us. Only plague, which does still occur—there was an epidemic in India in the 1990s, and it has regular outbreaks in Madagascar—has diminished in scope and ferocity. And new diseases are surely on the horizon. Thus, while much of this book is historical, it is not solely about history.

The connection between epidemics and pandemics and the growth of the modern state is clear. As early as the fifteenth century, in response to the plague, Italian city states formed state-sponsored boards of health. The cholera pandemics of the nineteenth century led to nationwide efforts at quarantine—efforts that could only be carried off by a central state. Measures such as compulsory vaccination also demonstrate this connection.

Epidemics and pandemics cannot occur without a dense and mobile population. None of these diseases emerged in pandemic form until humans had settled down to farm and begun trading with one another. Infectious diseases need to be transmitted from host to host to survive; that host must be susceptible. Smallpox remained such a killer among American Indians because it was able, over centuries, to find non-immune populations; once those populations diminished, the disease naturally declined. Trade and travel were well developed by the fourteenth century; the plague took advantage of this. TB exploded only when conditions allowed

5

it: the densely packed cities and workplaces of industrializing Europe in the eighteenth century. AIDS has relied on human mobility to move around the globe. When pandemic influenza spread around most of the planet in a matter of months in 1918, it could only have done so because of the newly built transportation and trade networks and the heightened mobility brought on by World War I. Human, animal, and insect movement are critical in the spread of epidemics and pandemics.

Finally, people—eyewitnesses, novelists, poets, memoirists, government bureaucrats, journalists, historians, anthropologists, epidemiologists, kings, queens, and presidents—have been writing about epidemics and pandemics for centuries, reflecting on what causes them, what might stop them, and how people have reacted to them. We have, collectively, accumulated an untold amount of source material of value not only to historians. We have accumulated a record of successes and failures that should be an aid to those working on epidemics and pandemics now.

Chapter 1
Plague

Plague. A word more freighted with meaning in the history of disease would be hard to find. It is a disease we now know to be caused by a bacillus, *Yersinia pestis*, transmitted by the bite of an infected flea—a flea seeking a human host after its animal host died. It first appeared in the sixth century CE when the first identifiable pandemic occurred during the Byzantine Empire. It is commonly called the Plague of Justinian after the eastern Roman emperor Justinian. Where it originated is uncertain—it possibly came from the interior of central Africa to Ethiopia and went on to Byzantium via well-established trade networks. But it might have come from Asia. We don't know. It first appeared in the historical record in 541 in the Egyptian port city of Pelusium. It took two years to travel the length and breadth of the Mediterranean, sparing no country along its coast, moving on to Persia in the east and the British Isles in the north.

Although precise demographic data does not exist, it is clear that the pandemic had devastating effects on mortality. John of Ephesus, in his *Ecclesiastical History*, detailed his encounter with the plague as he coincidentally traveled along its path from Constantinople to Alexandria and back through Palestine, Syria, and Asia Minor. He documented fallow fields, vineyards with grapes unpicked, animals gone feral, and people who spent their days digging graves. The Greek historian Procopius said that plague claimed ten thousand lives in Constantinople in a single day in 542. The "whole human race came near to being annihilated." Evagrius, another contemporary observer, thought the plague took three hundred thousand lives in the Byzantine capital. These numbers are impressionistic—an impression of deadly devastation. Procopius and other Greek observers of the plague familiar with earlier epidemics agreed that there had never been one like the Plague of Justinian. Pre-Islamic Arabic writers noted the novelty and reported that the plague had a major demographic effect on the eastern reaches of the Roman Empire. Early Islamic writers chronicled death on such a scale and at such a pace that it forced the abandonment of burial practices. When it finally reached mainland England in the mid-seventh century, Bede, in his *Ecclesiastical History*, lamented that plague's "sudden pestilence rag[ed] far and wide with fierce destruction...and carried off many throughout the length and breadth of Britain."

For more than two hundred years, beginning with the Plague of Justinian, more than a dozen separate epidemics visited parts of Europe and the Near East. By the end of the eighth century it was gone, perhaps no longer able to find susceptible human or rat hosts.

The plague's effects varied from place to place. On a grand scale, the effects of rural depopulation on the finances of the Byzantine Empire—effects gleaned from careful attention to numismatic, papyrological, and legal evidence—suggest that the first plague pandemic might have contributed to the downfall of the empire itself. By contrast, plague did not reach Britain until 664; it disappeared twenty-three years later. Its immediate impact—mass death, the emptying out of monasteries, the abandonment of villages—was shocking. Its long-term effects might well have been negligible. Northumbrian monastic life was hard hit by the plague in the 660s; two generations later it was thriving. Plague seems to have been no match for good land, royal power, and vast wealth. These conclusions are based on slivers of evidence, for when one tries to look beyond monasteries and into life more generally, documentation disappears.

The impact of the plague was keenly felt in the short and long term in Syria. Ships infested with plague arrived from Egypt in 542 at the ports of Gaza, Ashkelon, and Antioch. From there it traveled to Damascus, then spread south. We know from John of Ephesus that it was devastating. From then on, plague struck Syria every seven or so years between 541 and 749. In the short term, high mortality and mass flight left many places empty. Over the long term, repeated outbreaks had a deleterious effect on agricultural production and the populations of settled communities. The mobile lifestyle of Arabia prevented the plague from taking hold and in turn increased the power of nomadic populations. The continued fragility of agricultural production meant a reduction in crop-based taxes and the rise of a pastoral economy. So frequent was plague in Syria and so devastating were its effects by early Islamic times that Syria developed a reputation as a land riddled with plague. The impression stuck. By the medieval period Islamic Syria was well known as having had a long and disastrous experience with plague.

What we do not know about the first pandemic overshadows what we do. This may change as more sophisticated tools of analysis become available. Careful reading of textual sources can get us only so far. Historians will need to draw from disciplines such as zoology, archaeology, and molecular biology if the mysteries of the first pandemic are ever to be revealed.

Europe's apparently plague-free centuries came to an end in 1347 when plague returned and took with it up to half of the continent's population—perhaps more. When the first wave of the so-called second pandemic finally fled in 1353, it left in its wake a continent forever changed. After it reappeared in 1347 the plague regularly revisited much of Europe and the Islamic world. Its last European outbreak was in Russia in 1770. The second plague pandemic was not one event; it was a series of epidemics that varied in severity, scale, and scope. For decades, most scholars have believed that plague was introduced once from central Asia in the middle of the fourteenth century and then established a reservoir. Recent research into the correlation between changes in the climate in central Asia and epidemics of plague in Europe suggest that the old model might need revision. It is possible that plague came to Europe again and again. When the climate warmed, the central Asian gerbil population exploded and became a highly mobile, widespread host for fleas. The fleas would then jump to humans and domesticated animals, which would then transport them to Europe at a time of robust trade relations between Asia and European ports such as Dubrovnik.

Over the centuries Europeans adapted to the plague, even came to expect it, and developed ways of dealing with it. As a result, reactions to and consequences of plague in Florence in 1348 were different than they were for the 1665–66 plague in London, for example. Florence experienced a new and novel event; London, as cataclysmic as the plague might have been in the 1660s, experienced a familiar and increasingly well-understood disease. None of this was so during the first pandemic. No one was prepared; no one knew what was happening. It was novel and uniquely deadly. It was the Black Death.

For seven years plague swept across Europe, devastating the city and the countryside. It first appeared in the historical record in 1346 in the Black Sea port of Kaffa and spread inexorably across Europe. It demanded an explanation. How and why were so many people dying? The how was explained in several overlapping ways: providence, miasma, contagion, and individual susceptibility. As with cholera, these explanations—especially miasma and contagion—would dominate theories of disease transmission until nearly the end of the nineteenth century. During the Black Death—a time when the late medieval rediscovery of the writings of Galen and Hippocrates, via newly translated Arabic renderings of Greek and Latin texts, was in full flower, and the notion of bad air causing disease flourished—miasma and contagion were not as opposed to one another as they would become. People might become infected because of the miasmatic air seeping up out of the ground as rotting vegetable matter released its toxic gases. They would then be contagious and able to pass the disease on to others—especially those uniquely susceptible such as sinners and malcontents, the licentious and the gluttonous.

These earthly explanations for plague's path were subsumed in what most thought was the ultimate cause of the plague: God's wrath. Before plague reached him, Ralph of Shrewsbury, the bishop of Bath and Wells, implored his flock to pray. Toward the end of the summer of 1348 he wrote, "Since a catastrophic pestilence from the East has arrived in a neighboring kingdom, it is very much to be feared that unless we pray devoutly and incessantly, a similar pestilence will stretch its poisonous branches into this realm, and strike down and consume the inhabitants." Divine explanations were augmented by others. In one of the most detailed contemporary explanations, the masters of the faculty of medicine at Paris wrote in October 1348 that the "distant and first cause of this pestilence was and is the configuration of the heavens.... This conjunction, along with other earlier conjunctions and eclipses, by causing a deadly corruption of the air around us, signifies mortality and famines." When Jupiter and Mars, in particular, came together, this caused a "great pestilence in the air." Jupiter drew vapors out of the earth; Mars ignited them. But even with this scientific explanation, one driven by observation and theory and devoted to the notion that medicine played a role in controlling the disease, plague was still ultimately caused by God. "We must not overlook the fact that any pestilence proceeds from the divine will, and our advice can therefore only be to return humbly to God."

Many reacted in horror to the plague, as Giovanni Boccaccio so vividly documents in *The Decameron*. Based on Boccaccio's experience in Florence, *The Decameron* is an unparalleled literary representation of the plague's reception. Boccaccio was agnostic on the cause—it might have been the "influence of heavenly bodies," or it might have been "punishment signifying God's righteous anger at our iniquitous way of life." Whatever the cause, "in the face of its onrush, all the wisdom and ingenuity of man were unavailing.... All of the advice of physicians and all the power of medicine were profitless and unavailing."

The misery caused by plague led people to abandon the laws of God and man; there were few left alive to enforce them. Those outside the city without medical care or family or community to take care of them, Boccaccio wrote, died "more like animals than human beings." Never before had such a calamity struck. "The cruelty of heaven (and possibly, in some measure, also that of man) was so immense and so devastating that between March and July of the year in question...it is reliably thought that over a hundred thousand human lives were extinguished within the walls of the city of Florence." A French observer noted that half the population of Avignon perished; in Marseilles four out of five were dead. As the disease traveled through France, the "scale of the mortality [meant] that for fear of death men [did] not dare speak with anyone whose kinsmen or kinswoman has died, because it has often been observed that when one member of a family dies, almost all of the rest follow." Suspicion and fear were rampant: family members treated their sick like dogs; neighbors shunned one another. In city after city the dead were buried en masse in plague pits that were an affront to established burial rituals and, at least in the short term, suggest a breakdown of order. Helpless in the face of such death, many chose flight, but in the Muslim world running from God's will was considered blasphemous. Some searched for scapegoats. Mobs wiped out perhaps as many as one thousand Jewish communities across Europe.

Despite the helplessness many felt, cities such as Venice and Florence responded by creating sanitary commissions. To ensure that the air was pure, they enforced the cleaning of sewers and the collection of garbage. When it seemed clear plague was on its way to Florence, the city forbade those traveling from Genoa or Pisa from entering. When plague did arrive, sanitary regulations sought to effect the removal of all "putrid matter and infected persons, from which might arise or be induced a corruption of the air." These measures were largely ineffective. Plague came and it killed. It would be a century or more before anything remotely effective could be put in place—and by then the virulence of the plague had diminished anyway.

People who lived through the Black Death reacted in numerous ways: they tried to explain the catastrophe; they reeled in horror; they ran away; they blamed outsiders. What is more difficult to discern are the longer term effects of the Black Death on demography, the economy, social customs, culture, religion, and so forth. In the near term, the plague decimated a significant portion of the population—one recent estimate is that 60 percent of Europe perished. Population stayed low for a century, leading to labor shortages, higher wages combined with inflation, and the opening of more land. Depopulation changed, for a time, some aspects of the social and economic order. This is best documented in England. In 1349, at Eynsham Abbey, the dearth of laborers forced the abbot and the lord of the manor to enter into a new labor agreement with the tenants with far more favorable terms. In 1351, the unfree peasants on the estate of John de Vere, Earl of Oxford, were relieved of many of their obligations. On yet another estate, the royal manor of Drakelow in Cheshire, rents were lowered by a third "due," according to the accounting official, John de Wodhull, "to the effects of the pestilence. The tenants threatened to leave (which would have left the lord's tenements empty) unless they were granted such a remission, to last until the world improves and the tenements came to be worth more." Wages went up, but so too did the cost of almost all basic goods—a demand for labor based on scarcity also meant a scarcity of goods. In response to demands for lower rents and higher wages,

Parliament passed the Ordinance of Labourers in 1349 and the Statute of Labourers in 1351 to set wage limits, compel people to work, and punish those who disobeyed. Facing a severe labor shortage, the government acted swiftly against those who attempted to take advantage of the crisis.

That laws against seeking higher wages and lower rents were necessary suggests that in the immediate aftermath of the Black Death and in the subsequent decades of the fourteenth century there was a perceptible change in *mentalité*. Elite commentary on the (much maligned) behavior of the peasantry bears this out. They used their newfound surplus to purchase clothes not befitting their station in life; they also increasingly took up hunting—once the exclusive enclave of the rich.

The poet John Gower lamented the passing of the old ways: "The labourers of olden times were not accustomed to eat wheat bread; their bread was made of beans and of other corn, and their drink was water. Then cheese and milk were a feast to them; rarely had they any other feast than this. Their clothing was plain grey. Then was the world of such folk well-ordered in its estate." But now "our happy times of old have been rudely wiped out." Because "servants are now masters and masters are servants…the peasant pretends to imitate the ways of the freemen, and gives himself the appearance of him in his clothes." Sumptuary laws directed at the "outrageous and excessive apparel of divers people against their estate and degree" also suggest that peasant behavior was markedly changing. Lamentations for times past, when people knew their station in life, were common in the decades after the Black Death. Despite the presence of laws forbidding both demanding and paying excess wages, the practice was common: in the face of a continued labor shortage, made worse by subsequent epidemics in 1360–62 and 1369, there was often no other choice.

Laborers in Italy demanded higher wages, too. In Florence, the chronicler Matteo Villani noted that "serving girls and unskilled women with no experience in service and stable boys want at least 12 florins per year, and the most arrogant among them 18 or 24 florins per year, and so also nurses and minor artisans working with their hands three times or nearly the usual pay, and laborers on the land all want oxen and all seed, and want to work the best lands, and to abandon all others." That these demands were more than the disgruntled wishes of a few is clear when one sees the official responses: attempts to cap wages and force people to accept employment no matter the terms.

Though it is difficult to get a grasp on precisely how standards of living might have changed—the data is hard, if not impossible, to come by—it does seem likely that both men and women in the decades after the Black Death, ironically, were better off than their counterparts in the decades of want preceding the plague.

Europe's demographic decimation was a short-term shock. Within a century much of the continent's productivity and population rebounded and even flourished. But it would take nearly two hundred years for pre-plague population levels to be reestablished over much of the western Mediterranean; it would not happen in England until after 1600. Yet the population decline did not have a long-term adverse effect. One possible explanation is that the pre-pandemic population might have reached a Malthusian critical mass where resources had reached their carrying capacity. In this view, the Black Death, while a tragedy in the short term, was perhaps, viewed over a longer time horizon, beneficial. The well-documented increase in real wages across all of Europe in the century after the Black Death might best be explained by the increased premium on labor. Attributing changes in the economy and demography of such a large swath of space to a single cause, no matter how devastating, is not possible. Even generalizations are hard to make. Many changes may have already begun taking place: population was declining here and there; in many places, labor relations and land tenure were undergoing change before the Black Death—serfdom disappeared from Flanders and

Holland in the twelfth and thirteenth centuries with no assistance from the plague at all. But on the other hand, it is possible that the Black Death jumpstarted a century and more of technological innovation. Power-generating devices such as wind and water mills proliferated; firearms did too. Were these tools a response to the dearth of bodies in the wake of the plague? Possibly. What seems undeniable is that if the plague was not the singular cause of change, it certainly was an accelerant.

A catastrophe of such a scale left a mark on literature, art, and worship. In the wake of the plague we see an excess of piety in some places, as well as rebellion against the strictures of the church. Central European flagellants—religious devotees who publicly performed their unique form of piety by whipping themselves, among other things—began taking on the conventional roles of the clergy and professing that Christ was on his way to earth to put an end to oppression by taking from the rich and giving to the poor. A fascination with the macabre in artwork suggests a newfound awareness of the unpredictability of mortality. Universities expanded in the plague's aftermath—a dearth of priests and the consequent lapses in learning brought on by the plague inspired their founding. In England, grand cathedral construction gave way to building smaller, more modest churches.

In the decades and centuries after the Black Death, doctors gained more confidence, mortality declined, and governments began to take a more active role in managing the plague. People became accustomed to plague as it became a regular feature of life in many places. London suffered seventeen outbreaks between 1500 and 1665. For nearly three hundred years—1500 to 1720—not a year passed in France without plague. In Egypt, it appeared every eight to nine years, and in Syria-Palestine there appear to have been eighteen major epidemics between the Black Death and the Ottoman takeover in 1517. Its regularity and the fact that there was never again a brutal and shocking continent-wide conflagration as devastating as the Black Death meant that there was much less fear and very little scapegoating; in contrast to the innumerable attacks on Jews during the Black Death, during the next century there was only one, in Poland. The extreme shock of the Black Death did not return; plague became horrifyingly normal. Medical doctors and municipalities gained confidence in their ability to confront it. While no one knew just when or where plague would come—it possessed, as one historian has put it, an "inexplicable randomness"—a broad pattern did begin to reveal itself: first, it struck ports; it next moved inland, and then from the city to the country. In cities, it appeared in some neighborhoods and not others; it moved from house to house, seemingly at random. Patterns of behavior became discernible. Flight was common. So was an urge for self-preservation that meant, at times, a disregard for others. Generally speaking, governments remained intact, and plague did not spell the end of the social order. Official responses to plague—government-sponsored health boards, hospitals, and pest houses, as well as the machinery of quarantine—strengthened the state across much of early modern Europe.

Methods of control changed as doctors less and less understood the origins of the plague to be found in God's wrath or the alignment of the planets. They sought more earthly explanations and they tried to cure it. By the end of the fourteenth century, and increasingly in the fifteenth, doctors began to see the plague as beneficial to their practice. The wealth of clinical experience that came from experimenting with various cures is well documented in a new genre of writing that emerged in the late medieval period devoted to explain plague: the plague tractatus. Because some epidemics were comparatively minor, people had time to get to know the disease in less anxious and terrifying circumstances than would have been possible during a major epidemic. The newfound confidence led many to claim that they had surpassed ancient masters such as Hippocrates and Galen, asserting that these former authorities had no experience with the disease they themselves now mastered.

After the Black Death, loss of life on such a scale was not seen again. There were serious epidemics—up to 60 percent of the population of Genoa perished in 1656–57, and at least six other outbreaks took upwards of 30 percent of the populations of places such as Marseilles, Padua, and Milan. Mostly, mortality declined. The marked reduction in mortality very clearly corresponds with the newfound confidence in medicine. Some of this confidence surely came with new understandings of the disease such as the need for isolation of patients. But it is also possible that the disease itself was becoming less and less severe as populations built up some immunity.

The idea of contagion has a long history. It followed a twisted path from Galen, who developed a theory of contagious seeds, to the Renaissance; along the way it stopped in the Arabic world, where it gained little traction over miasma and God; it began to catch on in Europe in the sixteenth century. The notion that plague might be contagious appeared as early as the late fourteenth century. Just as the Black Death was wreaking havoc in the Mediterranean, the Arabic writer Ibn al-Khatib offered one of the clearest declarations in favor of contagion. His views were in stark contrast with the more common Muslim belief that God sent plague. Ibn al-Khatib wrote, "If it were asked, how do we submit to the theory of contagion, when already the divine law has refuted the notion of contagion, we will answer: The existence of contagion has been proved by experience, deduction, the senses, observations, and by unanimous reports, and these aforementioned categories are the demonstrations of proof."

The theory of contagion that began to emerge in early modern Europe was often accompanied by miasma. And God was still very much present. Some, like the English preacher Richard Leake, had no tolerance for earthly explanations. He intoned, "It was not infection of the air, distemperature in men's bodies, much less the malicious and devilish practice of witches, or yet blind fortune, or any other such imagined causes, which were the breeders of these evils, but the mass and multitude of our sins." Plague was God's punishment. In the tiny village of Monte Lupo, in the Tuscan hinterlands, plague arrived in the fall of 1630. Secular and religious officials battled over its causes and cures. Religious leaders, along with most of the townspeople, wanted to placate God with a religious procession. Secular health officials, believing that plague was contagious, attempted to restrict such public gatherings and isolate the sick and their families. Riotous violence ensued. In Spain and Italy such authors as Francisco Valles, Vetorre Trincavella, and Girolamo Fracastoro suggested that diseases like plague passed from person to person. As Valles put it in his commentary on Galen's *Epidemics,* "No contagion or disease can occur without the transmission of something from the already infected person to the person who is being infected. That is agreed, since every natural action occurs by contact....There are thus sent out seeds of contagion, which are some sort of defilements, from the sufferer to the person about to be affected by the contagion." But early modern views of contagion were very different than modern ones. Stephen Bradwell, an English commentator, writing in 1636, mixes contagion and miasma without compunction, for they are not, at this stage of explaining plague (and other diseases), mutually exclusive: as he wrote, "That which infecteth another with his own quality by touching it, whether the medium of the touch be corporeal or spiritual or an airy breath." The infectious agent was a "seminary tincture full of a venomous quality, that being very thin and spiritous mixeth itself with the air, and pierces the pores of the body."

The (incomplete) shift toward belief in contagion manifested itself in a move toward quarantine and isolation of both people and goods, travel restrictions, prohibitions on public gatherings such as religious processions, and a general increase of state power over the individual lives of the sick and suspected sick. In northern Italy, where these measures were pioneered, boards of health enforced laws regarding public health in times of plague. They had little effect; plague still came.

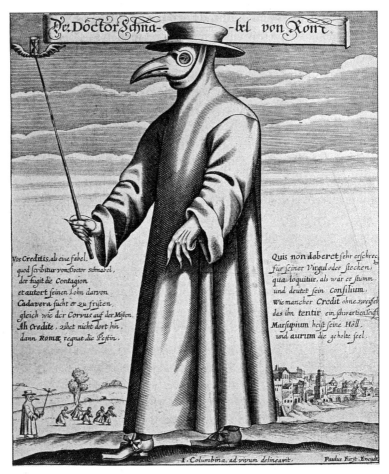

Ps. Doctor Schna-   -bel von Rom.

Vos Creditis, als eine fabel,
quod scribitur vom Doctor schnabel,
der fugit die Contagion
et autert seinen Lohn darvon.
Cadavera sucht er zu fristen,
gleich wie der Corvus auf der Misten.
Ah Credite, zihet nicht dort hin,
dann Romæ regnat die Pestin.

Quis non deberet sehr erschrec
für seiner Virgul oder stecken,
qua loquitur, als war er stumm,
und deutet sein consilium,
Wie mancher Credit ohne zweiffel
das ihm tentir ein schwartzen teuffel
Marsupium heist seine Höll,
und aurum die geholte seel.

I. Columbina, ad vivum delineavit.   Paulus Fürst. Excud.

1. **This 1656 engraving shows the iconic plague doctor wearing a protective mask filled with herbs to ward off the pestilence.**

What they might have reflected and reinforced, however, was an emerging association between poverty and disease. It did not go unnoticed in Italy, France, and England that plague preyed more upon the poor than the rich. Writing during the last major outbreak of plague in Marseilles in 1720, one doctor had this to say about a wealthy neighborhood: "The streets are wide, the houses are large, and inhabited chiefly by persons in a state of opulence and such are always the last attacked by a contagion, on account of the means they have to place themselves out of its reach." At a time when many thought plague was contagious and a disease of the poor, the wealthy began to worry increasingly about its passage between the classes. Plague became a social problem. It took on meaning as a symbol of the divide between rich and poor. Fear of the plague and fear of the poor went hand in hand.

Plague's contagious nature also had an effect on commerce as European states sought to impose quarantine on goods. Maritime quarantine dates back to the late fourteenth century, when it was first imposed in the port of Dubrovnik. Over time it became routine, if controversial and not necessarily effective. Quarantine was not relegated to goods alone; people, too, could be, and often were, detained. The association between trade, travel, and the plague was longstanding. Because most believed that plague had come from the east and that it was in some way infectious, detaining goods and people from that part of the world had an appeal that was hard to resist. The same was not so in the Muslim world, where contagion was far less well accepted, and the administrative capacity necessary for quarantine did not exist in the Ottoman Empire. India and China, other commonly invoked sources of plague, did not practice quarantine either. It was thus up to European states, particularly in the Mediterranean, to police their own borders. The sense that disease arrived from the east and the belief that nothing was being done to curtail its movement would only hasten the divide between east and west—a divide that would grow stronger during the cholera pandemics of the nineteenth century.

Not all states adopted quarantine with equal vigor. Those that did were in closer proximity to the sources of plague. Just as important was the growing association between a state's ability to govern and its ability to keep its people free from epidemics. This association was most powerfully felt in the independent Italian city-states and was in full flower by the late sixteenth century when all of Italy was engulfed by the plague in 1575–78. Italy's efforts to control plague through improved sanitation, strict control over the movement of people and goods—especially from outside—increased knowledge regarding the source of an epidemic, and the creation of more and more sanitary boards where there had been none initially made Italy unique. But its methods began to catch on elsewhere in Europe—Italy's influence is evident in England's first plague orders from 1578—and quarantine and isolation, especially, became more and more common.

Despite these early efforts at state control over epidemics, the effects were often tempered by lax enforcement, porous borders, and the power of merchants to subvert restrictions on their livelihood. Further, the Italian city-states were small, with populations that for centuries had been devoted to civic pride and protection. Erecting such an edifice in France, which was much larger and more heterogeneous, proved challenging. Even when maritime quarantine was in effect, as it was in 1664 in London as plague made its way from the Low Countries, it did not always work, for that year and into the next two London suffered its worst epidemic in more than a century. In theory, household quarantine of the sick was a good idea; in practice it did little: plague victims disregarded orders to stay put, and there were simply too many of them. Quarantine as a public health measure and its effect on commerce would come under considerable fire in the eighteenth century as it increasingly began to seem like a holdover from a less enlightened time.

If the beginning of the second plague pandemic can be dated rather precisely to 1347 and the arrival of the Black Death, the same cannot be said about the final years of the pandemic. It petered out slowly, leaving one place and then another, never to return. Plague visited England for the last time in 1665–66, when it killed eighty thousand Londoners. Half a century later it made its last appearance in western Europe in Marseilles. Fifty years after that Moscow hosted the last European epidemic. It visited

Egypt over and over again throughout the eighteenth century, killing as many as 20 percent of Cairo's population of three hundred thousand during the major epidemic of 1791. It persisted in the Ottoman Empire well into the nineteenth century. For more than three centuries plague had affected religious beliefs and theories of disease transmission, as well as demography and the economy; it ushered in the first state-sponsored public health measures. And then it was gone. When looked at across the early modern world, plague appears to have gradually petered out— after all, it was more than a century between London's last epidemic and Moscow's. But when looked at locally or at the country level, it appears to have disappeared suddenly. England had been visited by the plague regularly since the 1340s. Then it made one last dramatic appearance in 1665–66 and never returned. The same is true of France: after centuries in which no year was plague-free, the epidemic in Marseilles in 1720 was the last. What happened? Rats may have developed immunity, stopping plague in its tracks, or perhaps the dominant species of rat changed. Perhaps the climate fluctuations in central Asia that might have reintroduced plague time and again ceased. Further, despite the fact that in many cases quarantine was not effective, it might be that over the long term it worked to gradually slow down the movement of the plague. After 1666 England began to strictly enforce quarantine; plague never returned. But because plague lasted for so long in so many diverse places and ended at different times, it is not possible to determine a single cause of the disease's demise.

When pandemic plague reappeared in the 1890s, historical memory had not vanished. The nineteenth-century experience with pandemic cholera reminded those countries that experienced plague what it meant to deal with epidemic disease; most of the strategies deployed against cholera had been developed during the second plague pandemic. Its influence loomed large. And so, in turn, did experience with pandemic cholera influence the ways in which the third plague pandemic would be managed.

The third pandemic began in southern mainland China in 1890. That year, plague spread along the Canton River, reaching Guangdong and then southern China's largest trading city, Guangzhou. From there it traveled the short distance to Hong Kong and beyond. For the rest of the decade the third pandemic spread around much of the world, concentrated mostly in port cities. Cape Town, Sydney, Honolulu, and San Francisco all experienced plague. So did Rio de Janeiro and Buenos Aires. In Oporto, Portugal, maritime quarantine stopped the city's commercial activity. And while mortality in these cities was relatively low, fear and panic were high—eighty thousand fled Hong Kong; in Cape Town and Sydney quarantine became a means to put into effect racial policies designed to manage the black African and Chinese populations; harsh measures were directed at the Chinese in San Francisco and Honolulu. Plague made its way across much of northern and western India, where it killed nearly twelve million people. Senegal fell victim to the third pandemic in 1914, and for the next thirty years plague challenged French colonial management of the country. In Manchuria in northeast China a deadly form of pneumonic plague broke out in 1910.

The third plague pandemic was not the return of the Black Death. With the important exception of India, mortality was much lower—the disease might have been less virulent, and public health measures were more robust. Surveillance systems, maritime quarantines, isolation of victims—all of these and more were put in place, sometimes with brutality and heavy-handedness, to contain plague. In Alexandria, Egypt, rather than forcing people to adhere to strict public health measures, health officials enlisted local leaders to gain the trust and cooperation of the citizenry. As a result, mass panic was avoided, and Alexandria's epidemic burned out in a few months.

The pandemic's fast course around much of the globe was made possible by rapidly developing global trade networks and human

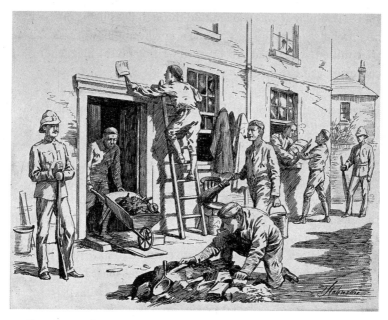

2. Convicts work to sanitize Cape Town during the third plague pandemic in 1891.

migration via ever faster steamships and an enormous increase in rail lines. The relationship between commerce, migration, and epidemic infectious disease—and the need to develop means of international cooperation to deal with the problem—had been evident throughout the nineteenth century as a result of pandemic cholera. The relationship became clearer when plague returned, and would be made so again in 1918 when pandemic influenza circled the globe.

Plague returned in the midst of the laboratory revolution. At the very beginning of the pandemic in 1894, Alexander Yersin, a Swiss-French scientist, and Shibasaburo Kitasato, a Japanese researcher, working independently, discovered the plague bacillus within ten days of each other. Next, as the pandemic made its way around the world, so too did the idea—first proposed by French scientist Paul-Louis Simond while working in Bombay in

1898—that plague was transmitted through fleas living on rats. Debates over who gets plague and why and how it was transmitted, which had preoccupied writing on the plague for centuries, came to an end.

Discovering the plague bacillus changed the identity of the disease. It did so in a very basic and rather sudden way: the plague that came back in the 1890s and was identified under the microscope in 1894 was a definite, knowable, if not quite tangible, thing; the disease that had been ravaging human populations since the sixth century had been unseeable and unknowable. After the identification of the bacillus this all changed, and the plague of the past turned into something identifiable in retrospect by its symptoms. Both Yersin and Kitasato claimed to have found the cause of the medieval plague. The modern, lab-based understanding of the disease would be imposed on the past. Before too long it was called *Yersinia pestis.*

The new way of seeing plague presented the problem of retrospective diagnosis. How can we know whether or not the disease that visited Constantinople in 542, Avignon in 1349, and London in 1665 was the same disease now known to be caused by *Yersinia pestis*? Some historians and biologists say they are not and stress possible differences in virulence; they claim that rats could not have traveled as fast as was necessary to spread the plague so quickly. They point to the absence of plague-like symptoms in some cases, and almost no evidence of mass rat death. Their case is built on differences between modern post-lab plague and premodern, pre-lab plague. The differences are stark enough that they cannot be the same disease.

Those who think that the two diseases are one and the same rely on similarities: the symptoms are the same, especially the presence of the telltale swelling in the armpits, groin, and the neck called buboes. It is almost certain that many, if not most, of the places that experienced plague in the past had considerable rat and flea populations. Like modern plague, plagues of the past—to the extent we can be certain—first made their way by sea, suggesting the agency of rats on ships. Also, supporters of the plague theory contend, the pathogen can change, and thus it is no surprise that plagues of the past looked different in some ways than the plague identified during the third pandemic. So what was the disease? By now, most historians, geneticists, and molecular biologists support the idea that the plague has always been *Y. pestis*. One reason for this is the emerging evidence from DNA sources originating in graves from antiquity, as well as from the late medieval and early modern periods.

Plague's relationship to commerce had of course been well known since its first appearance in the 1340s as a result of the Genoese trade with the east. From the 1850s to the end of the nineteenth century an emerging international community attempted to deal with the spread of infectious diseases at a series of regularly occurring International Sanitary Conferences. When the third plague pandemic arrived, scientific internationalism had reached an apex of sorts, exemplified by the International Sanitary Conference held in Venice in 1897, where the newest scientific knowledge about plague met a deep-seated desire for loose restrictions on trade. Science could serve commerce.

The Venice conference marked an unprecedented level of consensus on the part of the international community. The president of the London Epidemiological Society called the convention "a great advance on the part of the nationalities toward a truly *liberal* and truly *scientific* conception of the means to be adopted by respective governments for the prevention and control of infective diseases." Trying to contain the disease with quarantine fell by the wayside as more and more effective means of surveillance and reporting were put in place. If information about the plague's whereabouts was known, targeted responses such as immigration restrictions or port quarantines at the site of the outbreak could be launched rather than restrictive clampdowns inspired by fear and lack of knowledge. Not all nations adhered to the conference conventions—Portugal and Spain resorted to older, distinctly illiberal means such as ineffective military cordons around ports—but those that did, like Egypt, soon saw trade restrictions lifted. The consensus still held six years later, at a 1903 conference held in Paris. By then the focus had shifted to rats as the carrier of the disease, which in turn led to a focus on stopping plague at the ports of departure. This of course relied on both local capacity and interest in the two things most agreed were necessary to control plague: sanitary reform and a robust means of disease surveillance and notification. Across the world both of these policies were only unevenly in place.

The relationship between science and commerce was clear in India, far and away the country hardest hit during the third pandemic. From its arrival in Bombay in 1896, plague challenged the British colonial state's ability to manage the disease and called into question medical science's newfound confidence. The initial reaction was an unprecedented level of interference with and intervention into the daily lives of Indians, culminating in the 1897 Epidemic Diseases Act. The need to satisfy international demands that Britain stop plague from spreading to Europe gave colonial officials total power over shipboard inspections, neighborhood quarantines, restrictions on travel and religious gatherings, and sanitary measures. The act gave authorities license to try whatever they thought might work. This in turn gave medical science a newfound authority as colonial administrators allowed doctors and sanitary experts an unusual amount of influence over policy.

And those policies—fumigation and burning of houses; forcible removal to much feared hospitals where, among other things, caste conventions were not followed; forbidding funerary rituals; postmortem examinations; and the strict isolation of the sick—caused the greatest resistance to Western medicine in nineteenth-century Indian history.

The *Mahratta*, an English-language paper published in Pune, wrote that the British had never "interfered so largely and in such a systematic way with the domestic, social and religious habits of the people." One of the most hated practices, which spurred the most violent reactions, was family isolation, especially the removal of women to quarantine camps. In Pune, so resented was the practice of examining women in the streets and the frequent searching of houses by British soldiers that the plague commissioner, W. C. Rand, was assassinated in June 1897. The following year, after even more measures were put in place, resistance reached a head: rioting broke out all across northern India as a reaction to household searches, segregation, and hospitalization.

The colonial authorities were forced to relent—fighting the plague and the populace strained colonial capacities; the use of military force proved counterproductive. Perhaps working with rather than against the Indian population might be better. The sanitary commissioner came to realize that "experience is beginning to show that, what is medically desirable may be practically impossible, and politically dangerous."

After this change, even in Pune, where the most serious resistance had occurred, there emerged a spirit of cooperation between Indians and colonial officials. When the Indian Plague Commission issued a report in 1900, it noted that the shift from coercion to conciliation had been effective. What the resistance revealed and the new era of cooperation brought into stark relief was a lack of confidence in Western medicine, a realization that the British, despite their bluster, actually did not have the answers. Never again would they be able to impose their views on India in such a fashion. The suggestion that this was the dawn of an age of cooperation and equality would be belied by future developments in India. The point is that the British colonial authorities' initial handling of the plague revealed a state only capable of imposing its ideas by force. When that use of force backfired and the British were forced to come to terms with their failure, it was evident that the colonial state and Western medicine were not as powerful as they purported to be.

By World War I the third pandemic was either under control or burning out. But plague has not disappeared. Although it can now be treated with antibiotics, this must be done quickly, and because it is contagious it can spread fast. It has lingered for decades in parts of Africa and Asia; outbreaks in the 1990s in India and in the early twenty-first century in Madagascar remind the world that this ancient and feared disease still exists. But it has never again reached pandemic proportions.

Chapter 2
Smallpox

Until the World Health Organization declared the globe to be smallpox-free in 1980, it had been an endemic and pandemic disease for most of the last millennium, and possibly longer. Evidence from Egyptian mummies is tantalizing but not definitive; it is possible that the Plague of Athens, beginning in 430 BCE and so memorably described by Thucydides, was caused by smallpox. It has killed hundreds of millions of people. The earliest and clearest description of smallpox comes from the fourth-century Chinese alchemist Ho Kung, who wrote in what he called *Chou-hou pei-tsi fag* (Prescriptions for emergencies), "Recently there have been persons suffering from epidemic sores which attack the head, face and trunk. In a short time these sores spread all over the body. They have the appearance of hot boils containing some white matter. While some of these pustules are drying up a fresh crop appears." The most widespread description of the disease, which influenced clinical care into the seventeenth century, comes from the tenth century, when Rhazes, a Persian doctor based in Baghdad, wrote *A Treatise on the Small-Pox and Measles*. Evidence from China, India, and many parts of Africa demonstrates that smallpox has been a constant companion for centuries. Throughout much of northern India, especially in the eighteenth and nineteenth centuries, smallpox was considered a divine presence, not a disease. Sitala was the goddess of smallpox. The Cherokee, by the 1830s and perhaps sooner, had developed a dance called *itohvnv* designed to appease an evil spirit called Kosvkvskini thought to manifest in the form of smallpox. In West Africa, the Yoruba and others had a smallpox deity. In southern Africa, the Xhosa abandoned their funerary rites after a massive smallpox epidemic in the 1770s. No longer would they bury their dead; the infected died in the bush unattended. Death was no longer a natural, normal part of life but a feared and terrifying event. In Japan, the Ainu considered smallpox a god that transcended the boundary between the earthly and heavenly realms, turning people into ghosts who spread the disease among the living. It is no surprise that a disease that wreaked such havoc would have occupied a powerful place in the psyches of those it affected.

The African slave trade and settler colonialism brought smallpox to the New World, where it and other diseases reduced the indigenous population by as much as 90 percent. From the early sixteenth to the middle of the nineteenth century, as it continuously found a ready supply of susceptible hosts, smallpox caused a barrage of lethal epidemics across the hemisphere that morphed into a centuries-long pandemic.

Identifying the diseases present among the indigenous population of the Americas is challenging. Many sound similar, presenting with symptoms like fever, malaise, or a cough. Eyewitnesses could be maddeningly vague in their descriptions. However, because of smallpox's unique symptoms, most notably the pustules first described by Ho Chung, identifying it is less complicated than, for example, distinguishing between pneumonia and tuberculosis based solely on a colonial-era description. So clear were its symptoms to most contemporary observers—by the sixteenth and seventeenth centuries smallpox was a common childhood disease in much of Europe—that they called it by name rather than simply calling it a plague or a distemper. The Mexica had no word for a disease they had never seen before, but a description from 1520 in the Florentine Codex makes clear it was smallpox that had decimated the Aztec capital Tenochtitlán and allowed for the Spanish takeover:

> There came amongst us a great sickness, a general plague. It raged amongst us, killing vast numbers of people. It covered many all over with sores: on the face, on the head, on the chest, everywhere. It was devastating. Nobody could move himself, nor turn his head, nor flex any part of his body. The sores were so terrible that the victims could not lie face down, nor on their backs, nor move from one side to the other. And when they tried to move even a little, they cried out in agony. Many died of the disease, and many others died merely of hunger. They starved to death because there was no one left alive to care for them. Many had their faces ravaged; they were pockmarked, they were pitted for life. Others lost their sight, they became blind. The worst phase of this pestilence lasted 60 days, 60 days of horror.

There is usually no mistaking smallpox for something else (though separating it from measles can be challenging).

How did a disease like smallpox, which was not especially virulent in Europe until the late seventeenth century, become such a killer in the Americas? Colonists in early New England thought God had brought death and disease to Indians as both a punishment for their heathen ways and a mechanism to clear the land. The Pilgrim chronicler William Bradford, reflecting on a 1633 smallpox epidemic, wrote, "It pleased God to visit these Indians with a great sickness." As a result, "God hath hereby cleared our title to this place." In Roanoke, Virginia, Thomas Hariot reported that the Algonquian thought that "it was the work of God through our means, and that we by him might kill and slay whom we would without weapons." The Huron blamed the French. According to a Jesuit missionary writing in the wake of a massive smallpox epidemic in the late 1630s, the Huron considered the French to be the "greatest sorcerers on earth," because everywhere the Jesuits went, Hurons died and missionaries lived.

Historians often ascribe catastrophic population loss to what are called virgin soil epidemics. The concept is simple: a disease that for many years had been a common childhood ailment in Europe became a population leveler amongst people with no previous exposure. Virgin soil can perpetuate the notion that somehow genetics and race combine to create populations that are weaker or stronger. That is not so. All populations are virgin soil until they are afflicted with a given disease. Smallpox ravaged the Khoisan of South Africa in a virgin soil epidemic in 1713; in Iceland, between 1707 and 1709, an epidemic killed nearly a third of this "virgin" population. All the concept tells us is that when a disease like smallpox arrived in a population that had a large number of non-immunes—initially, everyone in the New World; the Khoisan in the early eighteenth century; and much of Iceland at a time when there had been decades between epidemics—it could have catastrophic results. Virgin soil is an appealing explanation for American Indian susceptibility to diseases like smallpox. But it should be used only to explain the initial susceptibility to diseases not previously encountered.

Other factors help to explain smallpox's destructive path. There is the possibility that American Indian genetic homogeneity after millennia of isolation left them susceptible. It is possible, too, that much New World smallpox was of African, not European, origin and perhaps more virulent. Smallpox's continuous reintroduction into the New World, combined with a time lag between epidemics, meant that in many places when a new epidemic arrived, immune survivors from the previous epidemic were dead. Many populations were not large enough for smallpox to become endemic, providing them no chance to acquire immunity. (This same phenomenon helps to explain the devastating effects of smallpox among the pastoral populations of Kenya in the early decades of the twentieth century.) As long as a sufficient number of non-immunes remained in a community, smallpox thrived. Pregnant women who had never been sick could not pass on protective antibodies; mothers could not care for sick children when they themselves became sick. Many Indian communities were densely populated; further, large groups often shared a single dwelling—perfect conditions for the rapid spread of smallpox. Without any idea of contagion, the well visited the sick. Flight was common; smallpox spread.

The disruption caused by so much death left many to die of hunger and dehydration. In the 1630s, William Bradford wrote of the survivors of a smallpox epidemic that "the condition of this people was so lamentable and they fell down so generally of this disease as they were in the end not able to help one another, nor not to make a fire nor to fetch a little water to drink, nor any to bury the dead." Smallpox epidemics were a product of other calamitous developments of colonization. The Great Southeastern Smallpox Epidemic of 1696–1700 was made possible only by the disruption and constant movement brought on by the native slave trade—a trade that for decades disrupted native communities via raiding and migration.

Smallpox rearranged the ethnic landscape of native North America. For more than a century beginning in the 1630s, smallpox, spread by the European/native trade in beaver pelts, guns, and alcohol, wrought changes in the Great Lakes and the plains/prairie borderlands. Devastated by smallpox in the 1630s, the Iroquois increased their "mourning wars"—the capture of enemies to replace Iroquois dead—against their longtime foe, the Huron. Smallpox ravaged the Iroquois; it nearly decimated the Huron. And this, combined with Iroquois military prowess, allowed the Iroquois to emerge as the dominant power. The same epidemic forced the Sauk and Fox to seek refuge further west among other groups, fostering the creation of new ethnic identities. Smallpox kept coming and coming, rearranging the ethnic order again and again. Differential mortality left some groups weak and others strong. The Anishinaabe-speaking Monsoni, powerful middlemen in the beaver trade by the 1670s, were nearly wiped out by smallpox in the 1730s; survivors drifted to other groups, and by the end of the century they ceased to be a discrete people. Into the void stepped people like the northern Ojibwa.

In the early 1780s, a pandemic swept north out of Mexico City, reaching all the way to Hudson Bay and the Pacific Northwest. On the southern plains, once the shock subsided, the Comanche avoided smallpox: rather than travel to smallpox-ridden trade centers, they stayed put and waited for trade to come to them. Among other reasons, avoiding smallpox allowed them to become the most powerful, and largest, Indian people in the American West from the eighteenth to the mid-nineteenth century. On the northern plains, the pandemic nearly wiped out the villages along the Missouri River. The Arikara fell by as much as 80 percent. In 1795, the French trader Jean-Baptiste Truteau wrote: "In ancient times the Ricara nation was very large; it counted thirty-two populous villages, now depopulated and almost entirely destroyed by smallpox, which broke out among them at different times. A few families only, from each of the villages, escaped."

The balance of power tipped toward the equestrian peoples of plains—particularly the western Sioux, spared the worst of the pandemic through the blessing of geography. By 1800, the entire Great Plains region was dominated by horse-mounted hunters. The Missouri River villages had been decimated. As William Clark noted when he and Meriwether Lewis visited the plains in November 1804, "Maney years ago they lived in Several Villages on the Missourie low down, the Smallpox destroyed the greater part of the nation and reduced them to one large Village and Some Small ones, all [the] nations before this maladey was affrd. [afraid] of them after they were reduced the Sioux and other Indians waged war, and killed a great maney, and they moved up the Missourie."

Smallpox continued to torment Indians into the nineteenth century. The Mandan, Hidatsa, and Arikara on the Missouri River suffered an epidemic that nearly finished them off in 1837–38; the same epidemic moved west, leveling the Blackfeet, the Gros

Ventre, and the Assiniboine. Coming to fill the void was the increasingly powerful alliance of the Lakota, Cheyenne, and Arapaho. As the expanding American people moved further and further west in the mid-nineteenth century, the Indian world they found, a world dominated by the Comanche, the Lakota, the Arapaho, and the Cheyenne, was a world created by smallpox.

In early modern Europe smallpox was a familiar foe, endemic in many places, flowering into epidemics and pandemics in others. Before the middle of the seventeenth century, smallpox was not an especially virulent killer. It was a low-level endemic disease rarely written about as dangerous in medical texts or the accounts of chroniclers and travelers. There were no major epidemics. In places like late-sixteenth-century London, few died of the disease, and those few were children. Then, somehow, smallpox changed. By the eighteenth century it had become the continent's major killer, surpassing the plague in the public imagination and mortality. Beginning in 1649, and recurring at regular intervals for the rest of the century, smallpox epidemics became responsible for more than 8 percent of annual deaths in London. By the middle of the eighteenth century that figure had doubled: in 1762 smallpox claimed 3,500 people and was responsible for 17 percent of London's mortality. By the end of the century smallpox claimed between 8 and 20 percent of the population.

Inoculation, and later vaccination, began to change that. Inoculation involved introducing a small amount of the disease into a cut to induce a low-level reaction. If all went well, the patient would experience a mild form of smallpox and would become immune for life, just as anyone who had caught disease and survived. Inoculation had been practiced in parts of Africa, India, and China long before it became common in Europe in the middle of the eighteenth century. News of its effects trickled into England and the United States at the beginning of the century—in Boston, Reverend Cotton Mather reported that one of his slaves from West Africa had told him that it was common; news of inoculation from China arrived in England in 1700; and word that peasants from Poland and Denmark were inoculating in the seventeenth century began to spread. It caught on in the 1720s after Lady Mary Wortley Montague, the wife of the British ambassador to Turkey, had her daughter inoculated in 1718 in Constantinople, where the practice was well-known; in 1721 her son was the first person in Britain to be inoculated. Royal inoculations soon followed, and it became a common feature of British medical practice.

There was opposition, however: worry that infecting people with smallpox was dangerous, and concern in religious quarters that it interfered with fate. Most objections met with fierce rebuttal: inoculation saved lives by increasing the number of those immune to the disease. By mid-century it had become firmly established across much of western Europe and the Americas. Improvements in method, combined with the inoculation of entire villages and towns rather than just individuals, had an increasing effect on public health over the last half of the eighteenth century. Big cities like London were much harder to inoculate than small rural towns; they continued to suffer from smallpox. Inoculation changed the way people saw smallpox: it became a disease that had a specific, efficacious tool to fight it with. This smoothed the way for one of the most important breakthroughs in medical history: vaccination.

In 1796, when Edward Jenner prevented smallpox in a young English boy by inoculating him with a small amount of cowpox, rather than human smallpox via variolation, it signaled the beginning of the end. (The term "vaccine" comes from Jenner, who called cowpox *variolae vaccinae*, or smallpox of the cow.) Two years later he announced his discovery to the world. While others had inoculated with cowpox before him, Jenner's innovation was *proving* that it worked by subsequently infecting a patient with smallpox and demonstrating immunity. Vaccination with attenuated cowpox was quickly accepted as superior to inoculation with smallpox: there was no risk of catching smallpox, which meant no risk of spreading it. Within three years of Jenner's announcement a hundred thousand people in England had been vaccinated. Millions more followed over the next two decades: two million in Russia and nearly the same number in France. By 1800 vaccination had arrived in North America; the following year it arrived in Baghdad, and from there it went to India. By mid-century, smallpox's ravages dwindled among American Indians. Vaccination with cowpox (and variolation before it with smallpox) helped reduce the death toll. By the 1830s, the Hudson's Bay Company had vaccinated good portions of the native population of western Canada; in Guatemala colonial doctors began to inoculate the Maya in the 1770s, even adopting Mayan medical techniques like the use of obsidian knives. In the United States, vaccination efforts among American Indians were generally too little, too late—hence the horrible epidemic on the Missouri. Even so, as more and more people acquired immunity and the disease was introduced less and less frequently, the death toll declined.

In Japan, vaccination initially received a skeptical, even hostile, reception from a country that was previously "closed." Those who imported vaccine to the country were in the vanguard of opening Japan to the West; vaccine was a principle conduit for modernity. By the 1850s vaccine had been accepted. The Tokugawa Shogunate attempted to use a state-sponsored vaccination campaign to help make the Ainu less "primitive" and more Japanese. Whether that project was entirely successful is debatable. But what is clear is that long-held Ainu beliefs regarding curing smallpox could no longer be maintained in the face of vaccine. A whole belief system was rendered ineffective in the face of this new and effective procedure. In Europe, despite some early opposition from those who thought the practice dirty or doubted the existence of a single disease organism able to be stopped by another, vaccination spread, especially as it became compulsory in some places. In Sweden there were twelve thousand smallpox deaths in 1800. In 1822 there were eleven.

The European population climbed as mortality from smallpox declined.

Despite the early success of vaccination, major smallpox epidemics still erupted on several occasions, for once vaccination had reduced smallpox to such low levels, the initial zeal wore off, and so did its effects: though no one knew it initially, vaccination did not necessarily confer lifelong immunity. Between 1836 and 1839 thirty thousand died from smallpox in England. The pandemic of 1870–75—sparked by the Franco-Prussian War—killed an estimated five hundred thousand people and snapped much of Europe out of its slumber. England and Germany passed compulsory vaccination laws. In England, however, debate over the cause of diseases—environment, contagion, miasma—along with a powerful distaste for state intrusion into English bodies and a sense that smallpox had diminished in importance led to vociferous and at times violent opposition to compulsory vaccination. Various provisions of the Vaccination Acts of 1885 were overturned in 1898 and 1907.

Despite complacency regarding vaccination and the regular appearance of local outbreaks, the 1870–75 European pandemic was the last major appearance of smallpox on the continent. Vaccination, as well as the gradual replacement of variola major by variola minor—which is less contagious and less severe—meant that by the mid-twentieth century smallpox ceased to be a major problem in Europe, the United States, and much of the rest of the developed world. When the US Public Health Service recommended abandoning routine vaccination in 1971, it was because more children were dying—six to eight per year—from vaccine-related complications than were perishing from smallpox.

Vaccination against smallpox was a monumental public health achievement. It is an intervention that targeted an individual's health *and* had a profound effect on the public's health. Reducing the number of susceptible people in a population to a number insufficient to allow an infectious disease to spread is the key to controlling it. Earlier measures geared toward the public's health, like the use of quarantine during times of plague, were very different. Quarantine aimed to stop the spread of the disease during a particular epidemic; vaccination reduced the possibility that an epidemic would occur in the first place. Once enough people had been vaccinated, smallpox, with no non-human host, had no place to go.

Smallpox is the only human infectious disease humans have eradicated. The last case of variola major was in Bangladesh in 1975; two years later variola minor made its last appearance, in Somalia. A little more than a decade after embarking on an intensified eradication campaign in 1967—something the World Health Organization had initially been reluctant to do, instead deciding to try to eradicate malaria and failing—the WHO declared the planet smallpox-free in 1980. By almost any measure—the cost; the logistical, political, and social challenges; and the humanitarian effects—it was a colossal accomplishment.

Alone among infectious diseases, smallpox was an ideal candidate for eradication. A freeze-dried vaccine had been developed in the late 1940s, which meant that the challenge of deploying vaccine in tropical climates had been theoretically surmounted. The telltale rash made it easy to spot. Isolation and surveillance, methods pioneered in the early 1970s by the WHO's Smallpox Eradication Program (SEP), worked to stem its spread. No animal reservoir existed. Unlike malaria, carried by mosquitoes, there was no vector to consider when contemplating eradication, obviating the need for large-scale environmental manipulation. The push for eradication garnered widespread international support, allowing the WHO to intensify its efforts—before the newly ramped-up campaign began in 1967 smallpox eradication existed, more or less, in name only; it was a poorly funded and inadequately staffed afterthought at the WHO.

But why eradication? Smallpox had been declining since the introduction of Jenner's vaccine. While still present in some countries, it was not the most pressing health problem in many places. Intensifying the focus on smallpox lessened the focus on the conditions that gave rise to diseases in the first place. In places where it was still present but not a significant concern, like much of Latin America, eradication seemed to some an unnecessary distraction from more serious health matters, as well as being an enormous financial burden. The United States alone spent $1 billion in today's dollars on the SEP. But it was the countries where the campaign took place that were responsible for the majority of the costs. Still, where it caused the most mortality, in parts of Africa and South Asia, smallpox claimed two million people per year.

Once the WHO launched the intensified campaign, progress was rapid. Within a few years the number of countries with endemic smallpox shrunk to four—India, Bangladesh, Pakistan, and Ethiopia. Smallpox was most intransigent in India, and that is where the WHO launched its largest campaign. Even there the SEP made rapid, though not necessarily smooth or conflict-free, progress. Coercion and intimidation fostered by the campaign's alliance with Indira Gandhi's authoritarian regime; friction between Indian authorities and the WHO, as well as between local officials and the Indian government; problems with supplies and the quality of vaccine—all these things and more made the campaign in India especially challenging. Still, by 1975 India was smallpox-free.

The SEP was a success. But it should not be remembered as the work of top-down planning emanating from Geneva. The campaign involved countless local people whose input was seen by all as essential; frequent international meetings helped to

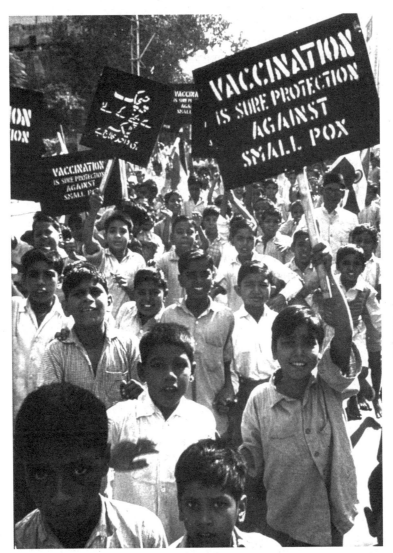

3. Indian children support the WHO and Indian government's Smallpox Eradication Program in the 1950s. Public acceptance of the effort was critical to its success.

encourage collaboration, share ideas, and learn from the myriad ways in which smallpox was and was not being controlled. To think of the smallpox campaign as successful solely because of the efforts of a few heroic individuals marshaling their troops or the work of the WHO would be a disservice to all those involved. It would provide a false lesson from the past, masking what the campaign really was: a multilevel, international, and indigenous effort that was responsive to often complex local conditions. Simplistic tales do no one any good.

Live smallpox now exists solely in secured labs, secreted away during the Cold War by the United States and the former Soviet Union. But in June 2014, two vials of viable smallpox DNA were found in an unused National Institutes of Health storage room, forgotten there for decades. This discovery briefly reminded the world of this once virulent, much feared killer.

Chapter 3
Malaria

Malaria originated in Africa and is caused by an infection with a parasitic protozoan of the genus *Plasmodium*. Throughout most of history, four types have infected humans: falciparum, malariae, ovale, and vivax. Recently, in Southeast Asia, as humans come into more and more frequent contact with primates due to deforestation, *P. knowlesi* has been causing malaria at an accelerating pace. The most common kinds are *P. falciparum* and *P. vivax*. *P. falciparum* is more lethal and dangerous. It is responsible for the vast majority of global malaria deaths.

Malaria might have existed in our hominid ancestors five million years ago. But because of the complicated lifecycle of the parasite, for an epidemic to occur a number of conditions must be met that provide the environment in which a sufficient number of mosquitoes and their human hosts can meet. Because it so often kills its host and does not live long in the human body—unlike tuberculosis, which can remain dormant for a lifetime after infection—malaria needs a constant resupply of hosts. This requires a dense population, which emerged slowly when the forests of central Africa began to be cleared for agriculture four to ten thousand years ago. Lots of mosquitoes are required. And mosquitoes need particular living conditions: those made available when farmers cut down vegetation and cleared the absorbent soil, creating pools of water ripe for mosquito breeding.

With few livestock available as hosts, mosquito species like *Anopheles gambiae* evolved to prefer humans for their blood meal. To spread, a malaria-experienced population must meet one that is immunologically naive.

Knowledge of malaria's early spread beyond Africa is scant. Solid evidence appears in much of the world after the first millennium BCE as malaria followed agriculture and human-induced environmental change. The region around Rome became malarious in the era of the late republic when economic conditions forced peasants to abandon low-lying farmlands, which then accumulated water and were transformed into marshy, malarial wetlands. Deforestation and the crumbling remains of a once vibrant drainage system added to the mix. From then until the middle of the twentieth century, southern Italy was malaria's European stronghold.

Malaria spread across early modern Europe alongside agricultural development. Its reach expanded during the era of the Atlantic slave trade from the late fifteenth century until the middle of the nineteenth century. It was during the seventeenth and eighteenth centuries, when the slave trade was at its height, that malaria from tropical Africa made its way into the New World tropics.

To thrive, malaria, like tuberculosis, needs human manipulation of the environment. Urban conditions gave rise to TB; those conditions that smoothed the way for malaria were largely rural and agricultural. The expansion of urban centers and agricultural production are related: the growth of cities fueled growth in agriculture. One can see this pattern in sixteenth- and seventeenth-century England, where a growing population and increased urbanization intensified agricultural production. In the Fenlands of southeastern England this led to draining some areas and creating marshes in others—conditions perfect for mosquitos and malaria. Malaria flourished as a steady influx of new peasant farmers provided susceptible human hosts.

Not all agricultural production is the same. Generally, where intensively capitalized agriculture took off—in the global north of the United States and parts of western Europe—agricultural improvement followed. In England, this meant ever more sophisticated methods for draining water, as well as out-migration of the rural population to cities, which reduced the number susceptible to malaria and capable of transmitting it. In the less developed global south, agricultural improvement was not as widespread; malarious conditions persisted; and a susceptible population remained.

Agricultural and rural development have been generally responsible for the proliferation of malaria, but poor urban sanitation and the presence of stagnant water can make malaria an urban disease—something that is happening more and more in the megacities of the global south. Other human-created environments also foster malaria. In the Panama Canal Zone in the early twentieth century, the mosquito most responsible for spreading malaria—*A. albimanus*—thrived in the conditions created by the canal's construction. An entomologist noted at the time: "*Anopheles albimanus* is closely associated with man and finds its most congenial surroundings about his habitations and in conditions he creates in the course of agricultural, engineering and other work." Joseph LePrince and A. J. Orenstein, authors of *Mosquito Control in Panama* (1916) noted that malaria "develops most rapidly when the soil is disturbed by large and extensive excavations and fills accompanied by the introduction of non-immune labor housed near the site of their work."

Following in the wake of agricultural settlement and the introduction of slavery, malaria wreaked havoc from the Chesapeake to the Mississippi valley to the Caribbean and beyond to South America. Exactly when malaria first arrived is unknown—perhaps early English settlers brought malaria (*P. vivax*) to the Chesapeake from southern England. By the middle of the seventeenth century African slaves had introduced

P. falciparum. It thrived among the non-immune settlers and their indentured servants across the New World tropics. When it seemed that enslaved Africans were less susceptible, they replaced indentured Europeans as a source of labor. The slave trade not only imported unfree labor into the Americas; it brought the epidemiological zone of tropical Africa to the New World.

Just as with cholera later in the nineteenth century and plague earlier, physicians in the tropics in the eighteenth century wondered if disease was a product of place or if it traveled. Many of these questions became tangled up with race and slavery. Noting different mortality rates, many wondered if Europeans were fated to die from tropical diseases while African slaves continued to resist them. It was a confounding question. As Dr. Robert Collins wrote of malaria and yellow fever in 1811 in his *Practical Rules for the Management of Negro Slaves in the Sugar Colonies*, "The reason why Negroes escape their fury, in the worst seasons, and most unhealthy situations, while whites die in great numbers, is a problem which no person has hitherto attempted to solve." Some argued that Europeans would adapt. In his classic text on the subject, *An Essay on the Diseases Incidental to Europeans in Hot Climates* (1786), James Lind wrote, "By length of time, the constitution of Europeans becomes seasoned to the East and West Indian climates.... Europeans, when thus habituated, are generally subject to as few diseases abroad, as those who reside at home." Did this mean there might be a universal human race, equally adaptable to the climates and diseases they lived among? Did climate determine biology? In the eighteenth century many thought the answer was yes.

Beginning in the nineteenth century, ideas about race began to change; the idea that climate determined health and that one would adapt began to disappear. Race became a fixed and hard boundary between peoples, and European optimism about settling the tropics was replaced by a set of rigid ideas about tropical places and "tropical races." In this way, malaria in the tropics contributed to the racialization of medicine.

After its initial appearance in the tropics in the seventeenth century, malaria was pushed ever inland via the varying forces of human migration. In the United States, an agricultural and malaria frontier moved west into the Ohio and Mississippi valleys. In Brazil, gold mining drew labor and malaria into the hinterlands. Massive forest clearing soon followed to make way for the vast farms needed to feed the new labor force—more than one million African slaves came to the interior during the so-called mining century of the 1700s. This new environment created the perfect habitat for one of *P. falciparum*'s most efficient vectors, *Anopheles darling*; the sedentary mining population provided the perfect hosts. Malaria exploded. But while malaria remained a problem into the twentieth century in the American South, the pattern established in places like England repeated itself: improvements in agriculture tended to reduce the burden of malaria, as these brought with them better housing and nutrition alongside decreased exposure. But in the tropics, malaria worsened and became a "natural" part of the region.

For much of the nineteenth century, malaria, along with cholera, was the quintessential miasmatic disease, brought on by the gases emitted from rotting remains of vegetable and animal waste; rain or other disturbances of the soil such as agricultural or urban development could contribute to the onset of these gaseous emissions. Its name even means bad air. Germ theory changed that. After Alphonse Laveran detected the malaria parasite in human blood in 1880 and continuing advances in the technology of pathology allowed more and more people to literally see, and thus accept, that malaria was caused by a protozoan, miasma theory no longer prevailed. Next came the vector. Near the end of the century, in 1898, Ronald Ross in India and Giovanni Grassi in Italy proved that anopheline mosquitoes transmitted malaria.

Malaria, like cholera and TB before it and plague shortly after, went from a disease explained by many things to a disease explained by one thing—the bite of an infected mosquito. The result: vector and parasite control, rather than mitigating the social or economic conditions that gave rise to malaria, prevailed.

Vector control worked—in places where mosquitoes were relentlessly attacked with sufficient resources or where the problem of malaria was limited. In the Panama Canal Zone at the turn of the twentieth century, William Gorgas, the colonel in charge of the United States' effort to render the Zone healthy, attacked malaria and yellow fever with unprecedented zeal by devoting himself to understanding the breeding habits and locales of mosquitoes and then destroying them. The abundant resources of the United States made this all possible. Within two years yellow fever disappeared. Malaria took longer—the reservoir of infection was greater, because it is possible to be reinfected with malaria (surviving yellow fever, by contrast, grants lifelong immunity). But malaria eventually succumbed.

Gorgas's success in Panama was a public health triumph lauded as an essential step toward the civilized settlement of the tropics. In "The Conquest of the Tropics for the White Race," published in 1909 in *Journal of the American Medical Association*, Gorgas considered the work he and others had done in Panama as the "earliest demonstration that the white man can flourish in the tropics and as the effective starting point of the effective settlement of these regions by the Caucasian." Optimism like this overturned the conviction that had prevailed throughout much of the nineteenth century that the tropics were unsuited to the white race.

The discoveries that led to the possibility of controlling malaria fostered a new field of medical inquiry—tropical medicine— devoted to understanding parasites and their vectors. Malaria led the way. According to tropical medicine's founder, Patrick

Manson, it was "by far the most important disease... in tropical pathology," because it was "the principal cause of morbidity and mortality in the tropics and sub-tropics." This new field spawned training programs, journals, and a research agenda. Schools of tropical medicine—the Liverpool School of Tropical Medicine was first, opening in 1897—were founded across Europe and the United States. A potent mix of optimism and hubris brought on by the very real breakthroughs in malaria control and the growing sense that diseases could be fought through modern medicine fueled the creation of tropical medicine. Malaria control was urgent, for in many places the disease was only getting worse as epidemics continued in the wake of uneven development.

Malaria declined where agricultural improvements reduced mosquito habitat and improved quality of life meant exposure to malaria was less frequent. But in many parts of the world peasant farmers had, and have, little opportunity to escape malaria and many chances to catch it. Peasant-based, undercapitalized farming left many people poor and continuously exposed. Large-scale plantation agriculture, focused on a single crop and employing the rural poor, often created the conditions for the spread of malaria: the destruction of forests for farms created perfect breeding grounds for mosquitoes. Since large plantations demanded lots of labor—labor not always available locally—a market in rural migratory labor emerged. Just as the forced labor migration of the Atlantic slave trade brought malaria to the New World tropics, labor migration in parts of Africa, South America, and Asia in the nineteenth and twentieth centuries introduced the disease into once malaria-free zones when workers recruited from areas with no malaria returned home and brought the disease with them. It was "the opening of the tropics" to large-scale, irrigation supported agriculture, according to C. A. Bentley and S. R. Christophers in their *The Causes of Blackwater Fever in the Duars* (1908), that turned malaria into an epidemic disease in India beginning in the 1860s. Where the soil drained poorly, irrigation canals became stagnant pools perfect for malaria breeding; the large tea estates attracted an enormous migrant labor force. It was the perfect scenario for spreading epidemic malaria.

Labor migration has been responsible for malaria epidemics at many times and in many places. For example, plagued by drought and left poor by sharecropping, the peasants of Brazil's semi-arid Sertão region—mostly malaria-free—migrated to the coast and to the Amazon for work. There they contracted malaria, brought it back home, and sparked outbreaks. An extended drought began in 1936, forcing greater and greater numbers of men to flee to find work. At the coast they confronted a virulent strain of malaria brought on by the recently introduced *A. gambiae*—accidentally imported by ship from West Africa. Those who survived the coastal epidemic returned to the Sertão, alongside migrants from the Amazon with still more malaria, and sparked a major malaria epidemic. The death toll was immense: officially five thousand, but likely more. A newspaper reported that the "human language is far from adequate to describe the desolation which existed in the region.... The general belief was that the Northeast would be depopulated because those who did not die at once would abandon it."

The arrival of *A. gambiae* combined with a susceptible population that was forced to migrate because of social and economic conditions caused the epidemic. In the 1920s and 1930s, likewise, forced migration of black South Africans from the malaria-free high veld into the malarious low veld created a new malarial population. And when they migrated back to the highlands to work on plantations set up by the very people who had displaced them, they brought malaria with them. With the spread of similar conditions showing no signs of stopping across much of the tropical world, a solution was necessary.

Those who wished to control malaria were split into two camps favoring different strategies: killing the mosquito vector or dealing with the infection from the plasmodium parasite. Gorgas's success in Panama and Cuba buoyed vector control, while controlling the parasite was made possible because of the discovery of the prophylactic quinine. Each had virtues and drawbacks. Quinine's limited value as a prophylactic was partly made up for by its therapeutic benefits. It worked to take care of symptoms, but supplies could be erratic and were expensive on a mass scale; its awful taste discouraged use. Plus, it did not stop transmission. That is, a person could be infected with the plasmodium, their symptoms stopped by quinine, but still able to spread the disease. Vector control worked. But it was expensive and logistically complicated. It demanded resources many places were unable to marshal. Neither addressed the underlying causes of malaria's continued presence.

After stunning success in several places, vector control prevailed. Gorgas might have been the pioneer, but there were other examples of successful vector control, such as the form known as species sanitation, which targeted specific *Anopheles* breeding grounds. Pioneered by Malcolm Watson in Malaya and then refined by N. R. Swellengrebel in Indonesia in the years just before World War I, this method of vector control was very effective. In Italy during the 1920s and 1930s, Mussolini's Fascist regime weakened malaria's grip by draining the Pontine Marshes, reclaiming them for agriculture, and resettling the area. In Palestine a smaller program of agricultural improvement and vector control brought malaria to its knees. And during the Great Depression in the United States, the Tennessee Valley Authority embarked on a program of rural betterment that involved ridding the region of malaria. Lowering water levels of dam-created reservoirs to desiccate *A. quadramaculatus*'s eggs, screening doors and windows (a practice more and more widespread since the nineteenth century), applying larvicides to breeding areas, and creating cattle grazing zones along shorelines to afford mosquitoes an alternative host all ensured the steady decline of malaria in the US South.

Vector control's place at the top of malaria mitigation efforts solidified in the years surrounding and including World War II. Breakthroughs in understanding the ecology of anopheline mosquitoes, especially increased knowledge about which species did and did not carry malaria; the success of Fred Soper and the Rockefeller Foundation at eradicating *A. gambiae* from Brazil; the discovery of the pesticide DDT during the war; and the same postwar impulse that spread TB control around the world all combined to make vector control triumphant. Malaria joined TB and smallpox as targets of the newly formed WHO's postwar global health agenda.

Malaria control was tied to the goal of fostering democracy and capitalism and stemming the tide of communism. The United States International Development Administration declared in 1956 that malaria control was easing urban overcrowding in Java and opening up Viet Minh–controlled areas to DDT spraying teams, and ridding the countryside of malaria in the Philippines meant that previously landless peasants could now become successful farmers on newly reclaimed land—and this in turn kept them from becoming Huk terrorists. Control of malaria meant the control of communism and the spread of democracy. The notion that "malaria blocks development"—that it meant the difference between becoming modern and economically well-developed or remaining poor and mired in tradition—was common. Malaria expert Paul Russell put it succinctly: malaria helped "to predispose a community to infection with political germs that can delay and destroy freedom." Biomedicine was for some, like American TB expert Walsh McDermott, the key to progressing in the modern world. "The biomedical goal of international development, or purposeful modernization, is to modify the disease pattern of an overly traditional society to a disease pattern that will not act as a major drag on a modernization effort."

So great was optimism surrounding the control of malaria that the WHO decided to eradicate it. Just as malaria became the archetypal tropical disease, it also became the disease that defined this era of hubris and overoptimism. Because of the abundant biomedical advances, especially antibiotics and DDT, it seemed like the time to think about ridding the world of some diseases. This was the climate in which infectious disease specialist T. Aidan Cockburn claimed in *Science* in 1961 that "we can look forward with confidence to a considerable degree of freedom from infectious diseases at a time not too distant in the future."

Malaria became a natural candidate for eradication. Knowing more and more about both mosquito breeding patterns and just which species transmitted malaria, having a demonstration of the power of eradication from Brazil, and being armed with an agent designed to kill the insect vector—all of these joined in the powerful postwar push into the developing world and added up to an unprecedented assault on malaria. Also important was that in 1955, when the WHO officially announced the Malaria Eradication Program (MEP), the global health bureaucracy was much smaller than it is today. The number of experts was comparatively tiny; many were like-minded; and most were members of the WHO's Expert Committee on Malaria. A very small group decided to eradicate malaria via indoor residual spraying with DDT. The major players were the WHO and donor governments like the United States; organizations such as UNICEF played important supporting roles. Funding largely came from the United States and such UN agencies as UNICEF; local governments covered the remaining amount—often at great sacrifice for what amounted in some cases to little gain.

The confidence with which the WHO embarked on the MEP was, it turned out, misplaced. Over the fourteen-year lifespan of the MEP, malaria proved far harder to eradicate in practice than theory suggested it should have been. After some early success in places like Venezuela, within a decade the program was faltering. Despite Africa having the vast majority of the world's malaria cases, the MEP, other than in a few demonstration projects, did

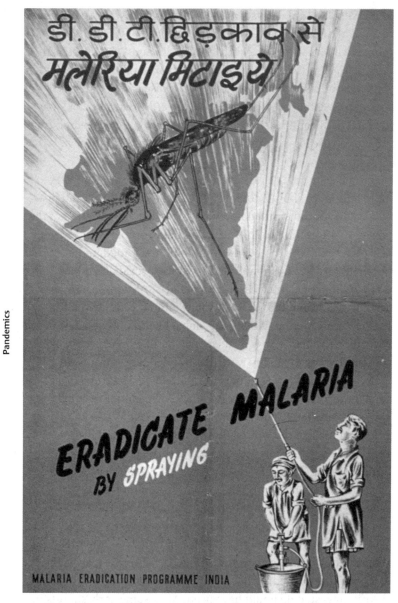

डी. डी. टी. छिड़काव से
मलेरिया मिटाइये

ERADICATE MALARIA
BY SPRAYING

MALARIA ERADICATION PROGRAMME INDIA

4. All over the world during the 1950s, the WHO's malaria eradication campaign was well publicized through commemorative stamps, posters (like the one here), radio campaigns, and other forms of propaganda.

not even attempt to rid it of malaria. The infrastructure was too weak and the problem too great; eradication on the continent would be impossible. So no one tried. In India the sheer size of the country, an unwieldy MEP staff of more than 150,000, the lack of basic healthcare throughout most of the country, and the growing problem of DDT resistance all added up to the conclusion that eradication was impossible.

In other places, like Brazil, the eradicationist impulse clashed with an already working program of malaria control. But the global health leadership at WHO, the Pan-American Health Organization, and the United States, as the major donor, remained wedded to eradication. In Brazil and Mexico, which were more or less forced to accept eradication, initial success with the program was met with later failures: when the MEP pulled out and mosquitoes (inevitably) returned, they were left with very little acquired immunity and no malaria control program. Then came resistance: first, by 1969 fifty-six mosquito species had developed resistance to DDT; next, as a result of careless mass administration, drug-resistant malaria developed especially chloroquine resistance.

The MEP did have some successes. Malaria disappeared from 39 percent of the countries enrolled in the program. Parts of the Caribbean and eastern Europe became malaria-free. Still, in 1969, when it was clear the program was not working, the WHO shut it down. Intense focus on a single, technological solution to the malaria problem while ignoring the sociopolitical context of the disease; growing concerns over DDT's safety, especially after Rachel Carson's *Silent Spring*; pesticide and anti-malarial drug resistance; lack of financial commitment—all of these help to explain the failure of the MEP.

Since the 1960s malaria has made a startling comeback. In some places where there had been significant progress in malaria control, like India and Brazil, there has been a resurgence. At the beginning of the 1960s India had under a hundred thousand cases; by 1965 they had jumped 150 percent, largely due to ineffective monitoring and follow-up in states with less robust health infrastructures; unreliable sources of DDT, as well as resistance, contributed too. In Africa, where malaria had never been under control, things got worse. In Zambia and Swaziland malaria surged because of new agricultural developments, HIV/AIDS, increasing poverty, and the eroding efficacy of pesticides and anti-malarial drugs. Increased population movements and a decrepit health infrastructure exacerbated the problem. Patterns of global economic development fostered growing economic inequality and massive debt, leaving fewer resources to combat malaria (and other diseases).

Malaria's resurgence has been met by another global approach to controlling the disease—the World Bank–sponsored Roll Back Malaria, begun in 1998. Roll Back Malaria, combined with the Global Fund for AIDS, Tuberculosis, and Malaria, has helped to draw attention to the disease, and this led to some increased funding. Yet malaria surges ahead. While not focused on eradication, and including Africa, Roll Back Malaria mirrors the MEP in some important ways. It has not taken into account what has been driving the resurgence in cases; it operated in places where the health infrastructure was weak; its efforts were not coordinated with other development work; and it has failed to take into account local conditions. While insecticide-treated bed nets, its key technology, have worked well in many places—the WHO claims they have been responsible for cutting malaria rates in half in Africa since 2000—they have also been repurposed, on a massive scale, as fishing nets in Nigeria, Mozambique, and elsewhere. Given the choice between fishing for food and using the nets for their intended purpose, millions are choosing food. The increase in fishing is having an adverse effect on fish stocks. A technology designed to help people stave off malaria is used instead to ward off hunger, but in the process the resultant overfishing is imperiling the very food source they rely on.

None of these programs focus on the conditions that give rise to malaria. The Gates Foundation directs much of its money to vaccine development; the foundation has also re-enlivened interest in eradication. And in May 2015, at the World Health Assembly, the WHO all but recommitted itself to eradicating malaria. A single-minded focus on one disease, however much the world would wish malaria gone, can have consequences. For example, although there has been success in reducing malaria in places like Zambia where it had been on the rise, it has recently been argued that this success has come at the expense of other types of health interventions. Focusing on a single disease like malaria can take resources away from programs that focus on general, overall health.

One of the greatest threats to malaria control is resistance. While resistance has been a concern since the advent of anti-malarials and insecticides, the problem has grown as it has been downplayed or more immediate problems held sway. Now artemisinin, long the most effective anti-malarial, is becoming less and less useful. At the beginning of the twenty-first century artemisinin resistance came to Cambodia; in early 2015 drug-resistant falciparum malaria had spread 1,500 miles—via human and vector migration—to the border between India and Myanmar. If artemisinin-resistant malaria spreads to Africa, the results will be catastrophic.

Finding a technological solution to the malaria problem, whether it be bed nets or more effective drugs, has been the dream of malaria control since the end of the nineteenth century; it is the central tenet at the heart of the gospel of control. The appeal is obvious. And by the middle of the twentieth century it seemed like all the pieces were in place to achieve what seemed the far easier goal of eliminating the vector via technology instead of eliminating, or mitigating, the conditions that help malaria flourish in the first place.

Chapter 4
Cholera

Cholera is a horrific disease acquired by ingesting water contaminated with infected fecal matter. Its symptoms—pallid, drawn skin; a gray and ghostlike appearance; rapid and often fatal evacuation of all bodily fluids—are shocking and appear quickly after infection with *Vibrio cholerae*. For centuries no one knew how to treat it. Then, in the 1960s, medical researchers and clinicians working in Bangladesh determined that a combination of salt, sugar, and water could replace the fluids lost to cholera (and diarrhea generally). Oral rehydration therapy has since saved millions of lives.

Though cholera had been present in India since at least the eighteenth century, the 1817 epidemic, because of its size and severity, is conventionally thought of as the beginning of cholera's history as a globetrotting pandemic disease. Since then seven cholera pandemics have traveled the globe. The first six were what is called "classical cholera" (*V. cholerae* O1). Each eventually petered out and cholera retreated to South Asia. For thirty-eight years, between 1923 and 1961, pandemic cholera disappeared. Then, for reasons still unknown, the El Tor biotype—named after its place of discovery in Egypt—began to replace classical cholera, and the ongoing seventh pandemic began.

Cholera, unlike tuberculosis, was not part of daily life; it appeared mysteriously, without warning, from the exotic and increasingly loathed and feared east. Its cause and cure were unknown. And as it became a disease of the urban poor and of immigrants from India and elsewhere, it came to symbolize filth and primitivism. Cholera exposed anxieties, revealed deep-seated divisions within medicine, and laid bare social and economic inequality in places such as Paris, London, Naples, and Hamburg.

While there are some themes in common—fear, debate over its causes and cures, horror over its symptoms and effects—each cholera pandemic has been different. The 1831–32 pandemic was far less severe in England than the 1848–49 pandemic—twice as many people died in the latter—but the public's reaction to it was far less panicked. The seventh pandemic—which we are in the midst of—has left Europe, where cholera has not appeared since 1911, unscathed. But it made its way in 2010 to Haiti, where it had not been seen for more than a century. Africa, which did not

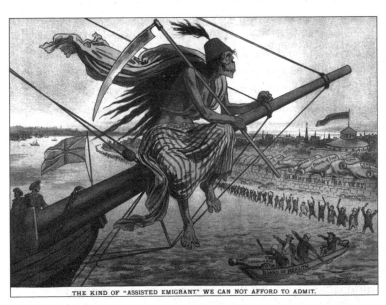

THE KIND OF "ASSISTED EMIGRANT" WE CAN NOT AFFORD TO ADMIT.

5. Fear of outsiders peaked during cholera epidemics. This 1883 cartoon shows an immigrant ship bearing cholera to America's shores.

confront severe cholera until the fourth pandemic in 1865–71, now suffers from more cholera than anywhere else.

The presence of cholera in one place and not another revealed to some observers essential differences between the clean and the modern, the filthy and premodern. A French writer, referring to what seemed to him to be a barbarian invasion from India, wrote in 1833, "There is reason to think that if the people of the banks of the Ganges had the good fortune to live under free governments they would tame the plague that their river is vomiting forth to poison other parts of the earth. The arm of liberty would snuff out the impure monster at its source."

Cholera symbolized a globe becoming smaller and more connected, its borders easily breached by the disease. The French delegate to the 1851 International Sanitary Conference noted:

Add now the communications between the peoples, today so numerous and more and more rapid; the navigation by steamship, the railways, and on top of that this happy tendency of the populations to visit each other, to mix, to merge, a tendency that seems to make of different peoples a sole and large family, and you will be forced to admit that for such a disease, so widespread and under these conditions, cordons and quarantines are not only powerless and useless, but they are, in the very great majority of cases, impossible.

Where did cholera come from? Beginning in the early 1830s, most thought the answer was India—Bengal, specifically—and Asia more broadly. Research into cholera's natural history in recent years has made its origins less certain—its protean nature, its clinical similarity to many other gastrointestinal ailments, its genomic instability, and its ability to flourish in marine environments worldwide suggest that the Asiatic cholera so confidently identified in the nineteenth century might not be exclusively Asian. This opens up the possibility that the cholera-like epidemics in Europe before 1817 were in fact cholera—a possibility shrugged off in the nineteenth century by those who could not imagine cholera having anything but an Indian origin.

The association of India with cholera has forever stigmatized that country. For reasons that are not entirely clear—perhaps this was a new strain; it might have been decades since cholera had broken out in India—the disease became especially virulent in 1817, leading to what a pair of East India Company physicians called, in 1819, "the most formidable and fatal diseases" to have "visited India in modern times." While estimates range, between 1817 and 1831 cholera likely killed millions of Indians, most of whom were poor and malnourished rural dwellers. Cholera spread across the entire continent, but Bengal was hit worst of all.

Cholera was more than a symbol of difference or of an interconnected globe. It was a physical presence. Its dramatic and sudden arrival in Europe in 1831 threw many into fits of fear; it signaled to some the arrival of a new plague. Some people fled, just as they had during plague epidemics; others stayed. Fear of cholera was at times out of proportion to the actual threat. In 1831, as cholera made its way through Russia, the anxious English awaited its arrival. Newspapers, pamphlets, and rumor spread fear of the disease. But Dr. James Johnson, editor of the *Medico-Chirurgical Review*, cautioned the press in a letter to *The Times*: "It will hardly be doubted that the terrible malady choleraphobia rages at this moment, epidemically, through every spot of the British Isles.... The choleraphobia will frighten to death a far greater number of Britons than the monster itself will ever destroy by his actual presence."

Seeing evidence of its destructive effects as it made its way across Russia toward Great Britain, a panicked writer warned in the *Quarterly Review*:

> We have witnessed in our days the birth of a new pestilence, which in the short space of fourteen years, has desolated the fairest

portions of the globe, and swept off at least fifty MILIONS of our race. It has mastered every variety of climate, surmounted every natural barrier, conquered every people. It has not, like the simoon, blasted life, and then passed away; the cholera, like the smallpox or the plague, takes root in the soil it has once possessed.

In Britain, in 1832, riots broke out in several locales. Coming on the heels of several well-publicized incidents of grave robbing, as well as one grisly and much talked about case of murder-for-corpse, the mobs directed their anger at doctors suspected of poisoning the poor in an effort to harvest bodies for medical school anatomy lessons. In France, some worried that the wealthy schemed to get rid of the poor with cholera. Cholera called into question the West's biological and cultural superiority: How could a disease from the primitive and backward East have the power to cripple the modern and progressive West? Cholera exposed horrific living conditions in the burgeoning metropolises of a rapidly industrializing Europe. Might it be that the very things making Europe modern were also those that caused cholera?

Misguided or not, fear matters. When cholera appeared in Naples in 1911, the Italian state so feared the potential consequences—reduced or halted trade and tourism; restrictions on emigration; the perception that Italy was not part of the modern, sanitary world—that news of the epidemic was hidden from the outside world.

Several of cholera's mysteries—mysteries it took most of the nineteenth century to answer and which were not limited to cholera—were especially important. Since not everyone suffered from it equally, many wondered why some got cholera and others did not. Was it contagious, as many by the 1830s believed smallpox and the plague to be? Did miasma cause it? Was it a combination of the two? To be a contagionist generally meant supporting such measures as quarantine. Those who believed in miasma thought quarantine useless; it was not people who transmitted the disease but the emanations of local effluvia—the rotting vegetable and animal matter in the soil and the bad air they produced. There was no strict divide between the two theories. Further, coming up with a sound theory was a challenge, because there was little methodological rationale for choosing some facts and not others; most tended to believe whatever suited their theory. A writer in *The Lancet* summed things up: "The progress of medicine, as an inductive science, is retarded by the construction of hypothetical theories, or the assumption of principles which are altogether gratuitous and imaginary, and also by the deduction of general principles or conclusions, from a limited number of facts."

While debates about cholera's route of transmission festered—and would for decades—something needed to be done in the short term. In this respect it seemed most were contagionists: from the liberal states like England and France to the autocratic ones such as Russia, Austria-Hungary, and Prussia, the initial response was to treat the disease based on historical experience with the plague and impose quarantine and restrictions on travel. States revived the practice of imposing a *cordon sanitaire* (sanitary border) in an attempt to keep cholera out; they kept careful tabs on the sick and the suspected sick, isolating them when possible; they blocked off infected zones; and they zealously disinfected, cleansed, and fumigated goods and people. As cholera approached Moscow in the fall of 1830, Russia mounted a vigorous defense—tearing up roads, destroying bridges, blocking passage into and out of the city. The military enforced restrictions on movement; disobedience meant death. Sixty thousand troops guarded two hundred miles of the eastern border. These severe measures were met with a mixture of indifference, fear, outrage, and resistance. Forced hospitalizations sparked popular unrest in Moscow and Saint Petersburg. In Vytegra, angry mobs freed patients held against their will; they destroyed hospitals.

The autocratic governments did not take a solely contagionist approach. They considered local conditions and instituted rudimentary sanitation measures—mostly toothless admonitions regarding hygiene—directed mostly at the poor. The possibility that cholera might have local causes, and the fact that it seemed to prey more upon the poor, suggested that the disease might not be just contagious. Growing ambivalence regarding cholera's method of transmission, popular displeasure at the severe restrictions placed upon daily life, and the merchant class's vehement opposition to quarantine and its effects on trade caused a shift to take place. As states, doctors, citizens, and public health officials gained more experience with the disease, the initial restrictions on trade and travel became increasingly difficult to enforce. Further, as evidence mounted that their effects were minimal, governments relaxed their approach. Additionally, as cholera traveled west along trade routes, the countries it entered drew on the experiences of those places that had already suffered—Russia, for example, had demonstrated that quarantine did not work. And thus, by the time the first wave of cholera in Europe was waning in the mid-1830s, belief in contagionism had waned. Fear of the disease, so strongly felt in the 1830s, never returned in the same degree. So different was the reaction to cholera when it came back in the 1840s and 1850s that places such as Lübeck and Hamburg in Germany adopted a policy of inaction; authorities worried more about the effects of trade restrictions and popular unrest than they did about cholera.

But once the initial shock of the first pandemic had worn off and the disease had retreated, reflection commenced. Relying on the historical experience with plague proved inadequate; alternative explanations and methods of control were necessary. The idea that it was strictly a contagious disease, passed from person to person, was cast aside. That it was a product of the local environment was not wholly satisfying either; not everyone in a given locale got it. Some believed that cholera was God's punishment for sloth and sin or brought on by its victims' immorality. Many began to notice an association between poverty and cholera. Living conditions might help to explain the disease's hold on some places and people.

The relationship between poverty and epidemic disease did not originate in the time of cholera; poverty and plague had long been linked. Yet in the 1820s and 1830s some began to probe the relationship in more detail. Louis-René Villermé's demographic research in Paris in the 1820s established that one's economic standing, and not environmental factors, explained the ill health of the residents of Paris's poorest *arrondissements*. Villermé's British counterpart, William Farr, revealed similar connections in the urban centers of England. Cholera appeared as the result of poverty brought on by the rapid industrialization and urbanization spreading across much of the West. This way of thinking could comfortably accommodate contagion and miasma. It could be that the poor lived in miasmatic conditions, perfect for the spread of an infection like cholera. Environmental explanations for cholera came to dominate.

It was in England where this view went furthest in fostering public action. The association between a given place and cholera (and ill health generally) was most heartily embraced by Edwin Chadwick, who in the 1830s was a bureaucrat managing Britain's Poor Laws. Fascinated with the relationship between poverty and illness and committed to the utilitarianism of philosopher Jeremy Bentham, Chadwick teamed up with several physicians and in 1842 published the *Report on the Sanitary Condition of the Labouring Population of Great Britain*. Replete with maps, charts, and statistics demonstrating the correlation between illness, poverty, and the sanitary conditions of specific neighborhoods, Chadwick's *Report* became the bible of the British sanitary movement, which reached its apex in 1848 with the passage of the Public Health Act and the creation of the General Board of Health. Villermé thought that an unjust economic system created stark differences between the rich and the poor; Chadwick, a committed miasmatist, only saw dirty and clean places. There was no need for large-scale social and economic restructuring; cities simply needed to clean themselves up. Chadwick and his allies advocated a system of water delivery and sewage that would constantly flush out miasmatic waste. Chadwick's vision, which would take a half century to fully implement, would be, along with Paris's sewer system, one of the great engineering feats of the nineteenth century. And while clean water certainly resulted in healthier cities, concerns over the health of the poor were not always, or even often, the primary driver behind the clamor for clean water. Consumer and industrial interests demanded it.

To most who cared to look, the connection between urbanization, squalid living conditions, and disease was clear. People like Chadwick believed that clean water would flush away miasma and the effluvia of daily life that caused deleterious living conditions. That it might be the water itself did not occur to him. But it did occur to John Snow during his pioneering epidemiological work in London during the 1854 cholera epidemic. Snow had begun thinking about the problem of cholera during the 1848 epidemic, publishing *On the Mode of Communication of Cholera* in 1849. Snow wondered if the feces of cholera victims were infiltrating the water supply. To Snow, cholera, unlike smallpox, was not transmitted directly from person to person through the air, since it was a disease in the gut and not the lungs. That cholera was waterborne was just a theory—a theory he would soon be able to test.

In a legendary feat of epidemiology, Snow mapped the location of cholera cases during the 1854 epidemic to determine where those who got sick got their water. The connection became clear: in Soho, Snow revealed, those with cholera all drank water from the same source, the Broad Street pump. After Snow successfully lobbied to have the pump handle removed, cholera cases fell precipitously. It was clear: something was in the water. But no one yet knew what it was.

In the 1860s, as the balance of opinion began to sway toward believing cholera to be a contagious disease, there were still those for whom miasma was the best explanation. In India, some thought the subcontinent was so plagued by the disease because it was in the soil, traveled by air, and preyed upon a weak population uniquely susceptible to its ravages. The Indian sanitary commissioner thought quarantining ships or putting up a *cordon sanitaire* to keep cholera from traveling "would be no more logical or effectual than it would be to post a line of sentries to stop the monsoon." But this way of seeing cholera was at odds with where medical opinion was headed.

The death knell for miasma, though it did not ring loudly at first, was Robert Koch's bacteriological work in 1883, during the fifth cholera pandemic. After isolating the anthrax and tuberculosis bacilli, Koch set to work on cholera. When Koch discovered the comma-shaped cholera bacterium *Vibrio cholerae* in contaminated water and determined that it must be present to cause the disease, the end of miasma was in sight.

Koch's and Snow's work did not meet with universal approval. Miasma, often in attenuated form, still held sway. The influential German hygienist Max von Pettenkofer continued to argue for a clean water supply, not because he thought cholera was waterborne but because cleanliness in general was the key to good health. Cholera came from the emissions of contaminated groundwater as the soil decayed. For a time, Pettenkofer's views had a powerful effect on German sanitation policy, influencing, for example, Hamburg's decision regarding whether or not to provide clean drinking water to the city's poorest citizens (they did not). When cholera came to Hamburg in 1892 and not to neighboring Altona, where there was a clean supply of drinking water, those who believed in the waterborne theory of transmission—which by then included most medical scientists and others concerned with cholera—were vindicated. But Pettenkofer remained firm. To prove his theory, he drank water containing the cholera bacillus and developed diarrhea—but not, according to him, full blown cholera. As he saw it, the X factor (the bacillus) was not enough in the absence of the locally specific hygienic and climatic conditions (the Y factor) to produce a locally borne infection (the Z factor). But by the time of his experiment, views such as his were rapidly losing influence.

Contagionism took hold at the same time as sea and land travel were becoming ever faster, bringing the "civilized" West into increasingly frequent contact with the "uncivilized" East and its diseases. Concerns about the spread of the disease led to an era of neo-quarantinism, medical inspection, restrictions on travel, and a heightened form of medical internationalism. The International Sanitary Conferences, begun in the 1850s, were called regularly thereafter as a way for nations to come together and discuss the increase in global travel and trade. They became increasingly concerned with disease, especially cholera transmitted during the pilgrimage to Mecca, after the pandemic of 1865.

In previous pandemics it took half a dozen years for cholera to travel from India to Europe. In 1865 it took just two, as rail lines and steamship routes linked the Mediterranean with the Red Sea. By the 1870s the conferences had become a forum for discussing restrictions on travel from the Middle East and India. The Italian delegate declared in 1872: "We have to stop that cursed traveller who lives in India, everyone knows it, from taking his trips; at least we have to stop its progress as closely as possible to its departure point." It was not just India: the entire East posed a threat to the West. As a writer in the *Times of India* put it in 1892: "The actual danger for Europe lies in the international Mahomedan places of pilgrimage Mecca, Medina, Kerbalah, Damascus, Jerusalem, the different places in Persia and the large places of rendezvous of the processions of pilgrims.... Oriental squalor and the absence of any, or any serious sanitary police at the great places of pilgrimage encourage the disease whose germ finds a fertile soil in the bodies of the pilgrims, weakened by all kinds of deprivations." The "stranglehold on the east," as Mark Harrison called it, relaxed over time as countries like Italy and Great Britain began to balk at restrictions on trade and travel in an increasingly competitive global market that demanded the unrestricted flow of people and goods. At the same time, the association of the East, especially India, with cholera has never disappeared.

By the early twentieth century cholera had become more or less a thing of the past in western Europe and the United States. Italy suffered an epidemic in 1911, and the country's robust efforts to hide evidence of it make clear how rare and unwelcome it had become in rapidly modernizing Europe. By the 1920s, the disease had firmly lodged itself in the developing world, and the north lost interest.

The seventh pandemic has had the greatest effect in Africa—90 percent of cases. As Myron Echenberg rightly notes, the African experience forces a question: Why is it that at a time when we know more and more about cholera and possess a cheap and effective therapy has the disease only grown worse and claimed more lives? For the same reasons that TB and malaria continue to plague much of the continent, so too does cholera: since the 1970s, lack of health infrastructure, increasingly fragile economies, growing inequality, and poor sanitation all explain cholera's staying power. War-related population movements have aided cholera's spread.

The seventh pandemic in general has been quite different than the previous six. It is affecting new areas or areas not touched in a long time, like the former Soviet Union and Latin America; it has traveled very fast; it has lasted longer than any previous pandemic—it has been going strong for forty years and shows no sign of going anywhere; and El Tor is less virulent than classical cholera, which allows it to travel more easily.

Cholera, more than any other infectious disease, is the product and symbol of social inequality. It simply does not exist where there's a reliably clean supply of water. Climate change will likely make this worse as cholera's reach will expand into those places most affected by and unable to mitigate the effects of rising sea temperatures—temperatures at which cholera can thrive.

Chapter 5
Tuberculosis

Tuberculosis, caused by *Mycobacterium tuberculosis*, might be the oldest human disease. It is part of a family of mycobacterial diseases, including *M. africanum, M. bovis*, and *M. cannetti*, that have been evolving for perhaps three hundred million years. The oldest fossil evidence for a tuberculosis-like disease comes from a five-hundred-thousand-year-old *Homo erectus* skull found in Turkey with TB-like lesions. *M. tuberculosis*—the type that affects humans—emerged in Africa about seventy thousand years ago. It accompanied modern humans on their migratory paths out of Africa, first across the Indian Ocean and then, some millennia later, into Eurasia. TB flourished when people settled down and began living together about ten thousand years ago. It has been with us ever since.

Tuberculosis affects almost all parts of the body—the bones, the blood, the brain. Its most common and deadly form, carried in tiny droplets through the air from person to person and highly infectious, is pulmonary tuberculosis. It thrives in densely packed places.

Like plague, it is an ancient disease and has been written about for nearly as long. Tuberculosis was also discussed in terms of contagion and miasma. Retrospective diagnosis is tough. TB can look like pneumonia or other respiratory ailments. Centuries-old descriptions of its symptoms—night sweats, weight loss, hacking cough—make definitive diagnoses difficult. TB was the disease that ushered in the laboratory revolution, for it was the mycobacteria that causes the disease that Robert Koch discovered under his microscope in 1882. A disease once known as consumption and phthisis, with unknown but likely myriad causes, became a single disease—tuberculosis—caused by a single entity.

TB did not rise up and suddenly snuff the life out of millions like plague; it worked slowly. No one thought it the wrath of God, divinely sent to rout sin and sinners. Unlike cholera, its symptoms are not especially dramatic. One is not suddenly overwhelmed with TB, dead or alive in a matter of hours after disgorging one's bodily fluids. TB works insidiously, initially unseen. TB did not inflame the press and public like cholera did in the nineteenth century, nor did it arouse people to massacre others as plague did. Yet TB was responsible for far more death than either of these diseases. As early as the seventeenth century, the Bills of Mortality— the early epidemiological records from London—indicate that 20 percent of deaths in the city were due to consumption.

The ways people once understood TB were quite different than how it is now understood. Richard Morton's comprehensive *Phthisiologia*, published first in Latin and then in English at the end of the seventeenth century, considered consumption in all its many forms. For instance, to Morton TB could variously occur when people swallowed nails and punctured their lungs or when women expended too much breast milk and taxed their blood, leading to a weak, phlegmatic condition. While these do not sound like modern TB, when Morton talks about the tubercles, those knotty swellings in the lungs, his descriptions sound similar to the disease we now call tuberculosis. Thomas Sydenham thought long journeys on horseback were the soundest medicine.

Across the eighteenth century, descriptions of TB became more and more specific. Italian and British anatomists revealed tubercles in just about every part of the body. Vague descriptions began to disappear in the early nineteenth century after René Laennec unified all of the pathological descriptions of tubercle diseases then circulating. Without the tubercle, he wrote, there was no tuberculosis. Making his observations possible was the instrument he invented for listening to the body's interior, the stethoscope. Whereas previously a doctor would diagnose TB by listening to a patient's history and observing symptoms, Laennec homed in on the tubercle, revealing it with his stethoscope and after death with an autopsy. There was a clear path between Laennec's stethoscope and Koch's microscope. Beginning with Laennec and other Paris physicians who also focused on single-disease organisms, TB came into focus as a single disease. It gained a name, tuberculosis, in 1839 when the Swiss professor of medicine J. L. Schoenlein unified all the ailments for which there were tubercles under that title. Koch confirmed it all with his microscope in 1882.

Although it did not inspire the same kind of panic or xenophobia as did cholera, TB did become the subject of literature and opera (most famously Verdi's *La Bohème*) and the tuberculous romantic poet (Keats comes readily to mind) occupied a peculiar place for a time in nineteenth-century European culture. Upper-class female beauty in the form of a pale, wilting woman who rarely saw the sun, preferring to languish for long hours indoors, was not dissimilar to the consumptive: pale, thin, and weak. As TB assumed a more prominent place in European mortality, so too did it come to occupy a more prominent place in various aspects of culture. The romanticization of tuberculosis was but a small, and short-lived, feature of the disease's history, overshadowed by its enormous effects on the lives of those whom it affected most—the urban poor. Yet the images of the romantic poet wracked by TB or the wan woman prone on her daybed have had remarkable staying power.

TB took a larger place in the culture at large, and occupied the nineteenth century's most prominent medical minds, because it had firmly lodged itself in the body of the public. It was the nineteenth century's greatest killer. It increased apace with industrial development and the growth of crowded, unhealthy cities like Paris and London. Marx and Engels wrote in 1862 that "consumption and other lung diseases among the working people are the necessary conditions to the existence of capital." So inextricable were industrialization, urbanization, and TB that by the 1930s these were seen as necessary steps on a country's path to modernity. As TB increased in Africa and India just before World War II, it came to be called a disease of civilization. In the late 1930s, Lyle Cummins, a British TB expert and frequent commentator on the disease in the colonies, wrote that India was then where England was at the "time of the invention of 'Spinning Jenny.'" Charles Wilcocks, a British doctor with considerable experience in East Africa, echoed Marx and Engels when he wrote, nearly a century after them, of the increasing amount of TB in the burgeoning urban centers of East Africa, that "there is little care for human dignity in the life that breeds these conditions, and men become, not so much individuals as units of production." TB had become symbolic of the harsh conditions of modernity— modernity exemplified by a rapid increase in urbanization, industrialization, and the creation of a laboring class.

What happened in the developing world in the twentieth century happened in Europe in the nineteenth. Records are hard to come by, but it seems clear that TB was Europe's leading cause of death. In western Europe during the first half of the nineteenth century, mortality rates ranged from 300 to 500 per 100,000. By way of comparison, today in the United States that figure is about 0.1 per 100,000. TB began to take its industrial-scale toll first in England, where an epidemic of the disease ravaged the working-class population from the end of the eighteenth until the middle of the nineteenth century, by which time TB routinely claimed fifty thousand people per year in England and Wales out of a population of eighteen million. In its worst year, Cholera killed forty thousand.

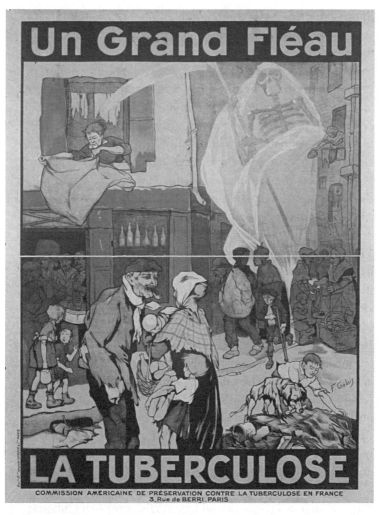

6. Slum conditions in European cities were conducive to the spread of tuberculosis. This 1917 poster shows a street scene from an impoverished area in Paris. The grim reaper is looming in the background.

While it is true that after about 1850 TB began a hundred-year decline, this does not mean the poor and working class were not still suffering from TB. They were, and disproportionately so. Once records began to be kept, they bore out what had been impressionistic. Postmortem examinations done in the 1880s at the London Hospital for Sick Children revealed that TB accounted for approximately 45 percent of mortality; 80 percent of these children were working-class. The same was true in Edinburgh: 39 percent of deaths at the Royal Hospital for Sick Children were due to TB; 98 percent of those children had been on public assistance. So great was the disease's impact in England that when it started to decline, so too did overall mortality. When one looks at France, Germany, Russia, or the United States, one sees similar patterns: growing industrialization accompanied by more and more TB. In the 1850s, in cities like Baltimore, Philadelphia, New Orleans, and Atlanta, TB was responsible for between 15 and 30 percent of all deaths. As it was across much of Europe, so too in America was TB the leading cause of death. Also like England and Wales, TB began to decline about mid-century. But the decline was uneven: it varied by location and social class; it also disproportionately affected racial minorities.

In the early spring of 1882, Robert Koch gave a talk in Berlin that stunned the world of medicine. He had identified the century's greatest killer, which he called the tubercle bacillus. The importance of Koch's work, its impact on medicine and public health, cannot be overstated. From then on TB had one single cause. Over time, the intense focus on the bacillus minimized, if not denied, the importance of the variety of social and economic causes of TB's prevalence among some populations and not others.

The notion that TB was caused by a single entity—the tubercle bacillus—did not catch on everywhere overnight, nor did it finally put to rest the debate between contagionists and anti-contagionists. Arthur Ransome, for one, was a prominent example of those who still clung to the view that diseases were not passed between people. Writing in 1887 in the *Transactions of the Epidemiological Society*, Ransome made what he considered a strong case for the soil being the agent. Though Ransome believed in the bacillus, to him, TB, like cholera, occurred in specific places;

it was not passed from one person to another. Ransome ascribed TB to fetid air: "It seems most probable, in fact, that for the active propagation of the disease, some increase in the virulence of the organism must take place outside the body, this intensification of its power being most commonly produced by the presence of animal organic matter in the air, in other words, by the absence of efficient ventilation. The favoring influence of a damp subsoil is also very distinct." However, by the early twentieth century most considered it contagious. In New York City, under health commissioner Herman Biggs, TB became an "infectious and communicable disease" in 1897, and a system of mandatory notification was put in place. Some states instituted compulsory hospitalization—a move some considered an assault on individual liberty for the public good.

The discovery of the cause of TB was cause for celebration—and overconfident predictions. The *Times* of London rejoiced at the likelihood that the "thousands of human lives which are now sacrificed every year to the diseases produced by the bacilli may at no distant period be protected against these formidable enemies." To great international fanfare, less than a decade after discovering the tubercle bacillus, Koch thought he had found a cure. But tuberculin, an extract of the tubercle bacillus that Koch hoped would act as a preventative, turned out to be useless as a cure (though quite effective as a diagnostic tool). Knowing the cause, it turned out, was only part of the solution to the problem.

Solutions to the TB problem included campaigns to outlaw spitting and attempts to build more adequate housing. One of the most popular and widespread treatments—and least effective—was sanatoriums. Part of the reasoning for the establishment of the first sanatorium, in the mountains of Silesia, was the belief that TB did not occur above certain altitudes. First appearing in Germany in 1859 and then popping up around northern Europe thereafter, the sanatorium craze came to the United States around the turn of the twentieth century. Designed to give patients a respite from busy city life and allow them to imbibe fresh country air, sanatoriums, it was hoped, would allow patients the time to heal. Absent an actual cure—no drugs and no vaccine existed yet—sanatoriums, in a way, harked back to a pre-Kochian view of the disease: they took people out of tuberculosis environments and put them into a healthy place.

Notions about altitude and TB changed, but the insistence on healthy outdoor living did not. In America, the cure for TB, advocated in such books as Lawrason Brown's 1916 *Rules for Recovery from Pulmonary Tuberculosis* and S. Adolphus Knopf's 1899 *Tuberculosis as a Disease of the Masses and How to Combat It*, was what came to be called the "outdoor life." Edward Trudeau most strenuously adopted the outdoor life at his sanatorium at Saranac Lake, New York, where patients braved the challenge of fierce winters by lounging outside in the hope that the fresh air would expunge TB from their lungs. Even though the relationship between cold fresh air and curing TB was unclear, even to its loudest boosters, Trudeau's sanatorium proved a great success: people came from far and wide to seek its cures. Philanthropy paid for the poor; the rich built their own cottages. Trudeau's sanatorium was private, but others were public. State or municipal governments, and in the case of American Indians the federal government, also ran sanatoriums. In the United Kingdom and much of western Europe, they were also run by the state. Many of them lacked the bucolic surroundings found at Saranac Lake, but they all emphasized rest, good diet, and plenty of time outside.

There were other attempts at a cure. The sanatorium treatment was essentially a passive affair; one mostly rested. Surgical solutions could not have been more different. The most common for pulmonary tuberculosis was collapse therapy, or artificial pneumothorax, which deflated the lung, allowing it to rest and heal. As Esmond Long, an American TB specialist, wrote in 1919, "The theory of artificial pneumothorax is simple enough…. [It is] the same as that back of bed rest or of lying, day in and day out, in a reclining 'cure chair,'—functional rest, enforced rest of the cured part [of the lung]." While Long was hesitant to go "too deeply into statistics," anecdotal evidence suggested it worked in what he called "desperate cases." The procedure surely had some positive effects in individual cases, but as a public health matter artificial pneumothorax was not a solution to the TB problem, nor were sanatoriums. Neither of these measures, as popular as they were, and as effective as they may have been in some cases, had any public health impact. Even when they were effective, they never served enough people.

TB demonstrably declined across the developed world, especially in the United States and Great Britain, between the middle of the nineteenth century and the era of antibiotics, thanks to specific public health measures and an improved standard of living. New public health departments in cities in the United States formed in part to combat tuberculosis. But no single cause can explain the overall reduction of TB in the general population. Segregating infectious cases in workhouses in Britain reduced TB in the general population by reducing the risk of infection. The same was true in New York: the identification and segregation of infectious cases by the newly formed public health department allowed for their removal from the general population to TB hospitals, thus reducing infection, and in this way sanatoriums had some effect. Reducing the risk of spreading infection was and is essential to stopping TB. But the resources necessary to do so have only been available in places where the standard of living has also increased. The absence of improved living conditions has been accompanied by an inability to reduce infections.

TB remained a disease of the poor. In New York, the large immigrant populations inhabited crowded, poorly ventilated buildings. TB rates there were far in excess of those in more well-off neighborhoods. In 1890, the Upper West Side of Manhattan had 49 cases per 100,000. In lower Manhattan, where vast numbers of immigrants lived, the rate was 776 per 100,000.

Tuberculosis

Between the wars, mortality for African American children under five was as much as 374 percent higher than for white children. Among African Americans in places like Baltimore, infections had not been reduced nor standards of living increased as they had for many sectors of the white population. Bureau of Indian Affairs prevalence surveys in the 1930s found that in the Southwest approximately 75 percent of the Native American population was infected. One hundred percent of Pimas over twenty tested positive. In Saskatchewan, 29 percent of all Indian deaths were from TB. Tuberculosis showed no signs of declining among marginalized populations in the US before antibiotics. But when Selman Waksman's lab discovered streptomycin in 1944 and ushered in the antibiotic era, it was as if a miracle had been performed: a formidable disease without a worthy foe had now met its killer. However, among the general population antibiotics killed off what was already dying.

As TB declined in the general population in the developed world, it increased elsewhere. Surveys in many places—among the Maoris in New Zealand and American Indians and First Nations in the United States and Canada, and in East Africa and South Africa—revealed alarmingly high TB rates. By World War II, it had become, according to health officials in Kenya, the colony's leading cause of death. Precise numbers were hard to come by, but the survey work, an increasing interest in collecting health data, and anecdotal evidence all made clear that TB was on the rise in much of Asia and Africa and among indigenous populations in the Americas.

For a time, a variety of racial explanations dominated the debate over why TB was increasing. Peoples in the less developed parts of the world—the "native races"—were virgin soil for TB; they were uniquely racially susceptible; or they had not become "tubercularized." Black South Africans, American Indians, and African Americans were most frequently the objects of this way of thinking. In India race-based explanations had little purchase, but evolutionary ideas concerning civilization did. In 1933, the public health commissioner of Bombay expressed a widespread belief about modernization, industrialization, and urbanization in India:

> Most western countries are said to have already passed through the epidemic stage…but it is difficult to state exactly at what stage the disease is now in India. Some hold that the peak has not yet been reached, that India is still in the early stages, and that the extent of tuberculinisation of the population is midway between that of the African races and the highly industrialised and urbanised European races. This view may or may not be correct but the fact is that the disease is rampant.

Racial ideas were powerful, but not irrefutable. At the end of the 1930s, as more and more data became available, they began to crumble. In Tanganyika, British TB expert Charles Wilcocks determined through an extensive X-ray survey that black Africans had in fact been resisting TB all along; healed lesions proved it. (Similar research among American Indians simultaneously showed the same thing.) Wilcocks knew that his finding was of more than "theoretical interest." His research would give "ground for the hope that adequate treatment can be made effective, and that the alteration in the conditions of life and education, which is the subject of all public health work, can help to control tuberculosis." As a result of work like Wilcocks's and generally changing ideas about race, by the end of World War II most TB workers had abandoned racial reasoning. TB was a disease of poverty. But while racial explanations may have been eradicated, TB had not been.

Before World War II little had been done to combat TB among the world's marginalized. But then, very quickly, several developments came together to inaugurate what was the most productive time in TB control the world had yet seen. The formation of postwar UN agencies like the World Health Organization (WHO) and UNICEF was part and parcel of the postwar impulse—an impulse sparked by a variety of motivations such as Cold War competition for hearts and minds, humanitarianism, and economic interest in new labor and consumer markets—to develop what came to be called the Third World. Combined with the recent discovery of antibiotics that actually cured TB and the positive results from the large-scale American Indian trial of the BCG vaccine (bacillus Calmette-Guérin—named for the two French biologists who developed it in 1908), the time was ripe to tackle TB in the developing world. In 1953 the WHO, referring to its planned mass BCG vaccine campaign, was prepared to launch what it called the "largest mass action the world has ever known against one single disease." By the end of the 1950s the sense that biomedical technology could finally solve the TB problem was palpable. As the WHO put it in 1958: "The possibilities for developing a tuberculosis control programme based on measures which, when applied in a public health programme, will prove effective, acceptable to the population, and not too expensive for use on a mass scale, are today, for the first time in history, really very great. The two main elements in this programme are vaccination and the use of the anti-tuberculosis drugs."

BCG made its way around the world into tens of millions of bodies, and antibiotics showed extraordinary promise. But the challenge was enormous. Hope mixed with despair in the world of TB control—despair over conflicting reports on BCG's efficacy and serious problems getting antibiotics to work as well in the real world as they had in trials. Testing BCG and antibiotics became the focus of much of the work of the WHO, UNICEF, and the British Medical Research Council (MRC), especially in India and Kenya. Vaccination held great promise because it would prevent TB; antibiotics offered a cure. But BCG's efficacy ranged considerably. Before the war, there was anecdotal evidence of its value from the French and Belgian colonies, where it had been used extensively. In 1946, results from a controlled trial seemed to demonstrate that it worked well among American Indians. Yet, as it spread around the globe, it was proving to be less than promising. Then, in 1979, the results of the largest trial to date appeared. BCG had 0 percent efficacy among 360,000 south Indian test subjects. Why its efficacy has ranged so widely has never been adequately explained. Differing strains of vaccine, exposure to environmental mycobacteria, high rates of infection, exposure to sunlight adversely affecting BCG—all these explanations and more have been offered. What kept BCG going for so many decades was the hope that it would work and the very powerful sense that no other preventative existed.

Antibiotics incontrovertibly worked. But they were frequently rolled out in places unable to effectively manage them; supplies ran low; some drug combinations were expensive, toxic, and/or difficult to administer. Facing these challenges, researchers from the WHO and the MRC developed cheaper drug regimens and demonstrated that self-administration in the home was possible. But all the energy, expertise, and breakthroughs could not combat what became in some places a serious, at times insurmountable, problem: drug resistance. In less than a decade, Kenya went from having no antibiotics at all to facing a nearly uncontrollable epidemic of drug-resistant TB by the mid-1960s. The same was true in other places where antibiotics existed in the absence of an effective management system. For decades, the WHO and others ignored the problem or downplayed its seriousness.

The postwar assault on TB joined the simultaneous push to eradicate malaria (unsuccessfully) and smallpox (successfully) as a narrowly conceived biomedical solution to disease control. For TB, this was never enough. Critiques of this approach, like the robust resistance movement against the mass BCG campaign in India in the 1950s, were very rarely taken seriously. In India and elsewhere, the notion that improving living standards was the key to lowering rates of TB was all well and good, but it was unrealistic, most in the development business thought. Many more agreed with American TB expert Walsh McDermott, who argued that because of advances in biomedicine, TB was a "disease

[that] can be decisively altered *without* having to await improvement in the social infrastructure."

By the mid-1970s, innovation and energy in global TB control had disappeared. TB was a neglected disease. But it had not gone away. And those still left working on TB, as well as those who continued to be at risk of contracting it, faced their biggest challenge yet: HIV/AIDS.

Because HIV weakens the immune system, it is the perfect companion for TB. It leaves those who are HIV-positive more susceptible to becoming infected with TB, and it is very effective at allowing a latent TB infection to fluoresce into an active one. In 1987 two researchers wrote that the "combination of both diseases could be at the root of a horrifying hecatomb [sacrifice or slaughter of many victims] in the years to come." So serious was the problem that in 1994 the WHO and the International Union against Tuberculosis and Lung Disease warned that the "combined epidemics of HIV and tuberculosis present a public health challenge unlike any other faced this century." Despite the early recognition of the relationship between the two diseases, very little was done during the first three decades of the HIV pandemic to stem the tide of HIV/TB. Renowned TB and HIV expert Anthony Harries, along with several colleagues, thundered in 2010 that the response to TB/HIV had been "timid, slow, and uncoordinated. If this situation had been a war...our efforts would have been ridiculed as half-hearted and ineffectual." Sub-Saharan Africa has been hit worst of all. Largely as a result of its deadly companion, TB went from a prevalence rate of 146 per 100,000 in 1990 to 345 per 100,000 in 2003. TB is now the number one killer of those with HIV/AIDS. For decades a combination of factors conspired to allow the co-pandemic to flourish: global indifference to TB by the end of the 1970s, the appearance of a new disease teaming up with an old one, the early neglect of HIV/AIDS in Africa, and continued incoherence and lack of leadership on global AIDS.

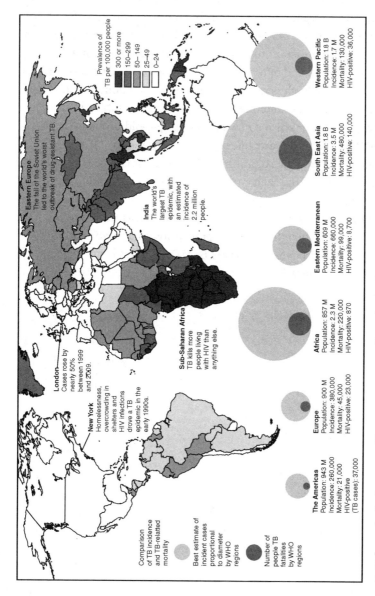

7. **Tuberculosis does not affect everyone equally. It is much more prevalent in some places than others.**

Added to the HIV/TB pandemic is the ever growing multi-drug-resistant (MDR) TB problem. Often billed as a new scourge, it is actually a continuation of the problem first encountered in places like Kenya in the 1950s and 1960s, only now it is worse. MDR-TB sufferers are resistant to at least isoniazid and rifampin, the two most common and effective antibiotics. Extensively drug-resistant (XDR) TB—which is resistant to isoniazid or rifampin and at least one of the fluoroquinolones and one of the injectable drugs—while new on its face, is also a new face of the age-old problem. Both MDR and XDR-TB are, like simple drug-resistant TB before them, a consequence of antibiotics being mismanaged at all levels: patients not taking their drugs; poor infection control; drug shortages; derelict program administration; the insistence, at times, that drug-resistant TB is simply not a big deal; and the more recent, though changing, perception that treating MDR-TB is not cost-effective. Like HIV/TB, MDR-TB has been neglected. Tuberculosis now kills more people than at any other time in history.

Chapter 6
Influenza

The influenza that swept across the globe in two waves in 1918 and a third in 1919 was the worst pandemic in history since the Black Death. Influenza had erupted into pandemic form before— most recently, and severely, in 1889–1892. But none approached the impact of the World War I era pandemic. It killed at least fifty million people. Most of that death came during the apocalyptic months of October and November. Looking back, the *British Medical Journal* wrote in April 1919 that in Bombay influenza "caused a havoc to which the Black Death...alone affords a parallel." It is still not known where the virus originated. Asia has often been cited. In Italy, rumors spread that it was not flu at all; it was chemical warfare perpetrated by the Germans. A pamphlet by an Italian doctor asked the question in its title: "Are the Latest Serious Epidemics of Criminal Origin?" The first known outbreak was at Camp Funston, Kansas, on March 5, 1918. From there it traveled to other forts and military facilities. It boarded ships bound for France in April. It spread quickly across Europe, reaching North Africa and India, and then going on to China and Australia by July. Flu struck so many longshoremen in the Philippines that dock work ground to a halt. The pandemic traveled the globe in four months.

The second, far more deadly, wave began in France in August 1918. It raced across the world via maritime trade and troop transport, appearing simultaneously in Boston; Brest, France; and Freetown, Sierra Leone. The Trans-Siberian Railroad carried it into northern Asia. Indian and British troops brought it to Iran, where it killed between 10 and 25 percent of the war- and famine-ravaged population. It arrived in Japan onboard a ship from the Siberian port city of Vladivostok, then under Japanese occupation. After it landed on the west coast of Africa, in Freetown—where the newspapers reported that the country "is all upside down...people are dying like rats....the dead are now buried in trenches because of a lack of room in the cemeteries"—it made its way into the interior via newly opened rail lines. It came to Ghana without warning. A colonial official noted that in the north "Lorha is like a deserted village, one sees no one. I hear that some Lobis are wondering if this is the end of the world." Once it arrived in Cape Town, it quickly made its way north via railroad. Flu's spread across South Africa was swift, as the nation had one of the continent's busiest ports and the most well-developed internal transportation networks. It followed the Congo River aboard steamship almost back to the Atlantic Coast. Flu came to the other side of Africa via the Indian Ocean trade, first appearing in Mombasa in late September.

Within a few months the second wave had washed over nearly every inhabited place on the planet. The milder third wave arrived in the winter of 1919 and was gone by the spring. The pandemic was over.

The demographic effects were staggering. Half a billion people—a third of the world's population—were infected. Incomplete reporting and inaccurate diagnosis make coming up with a precise death toll impossible. In many of the places hardest hit, such as India and sub-Saharan Africa, demographic data were scanty, and the limited medical personnel kept few records. China, where the pandemic likely had devastating effects, did not begin keeping records until the 1930s. Given the virulence of the disease, actual mortality was certainly greater than the reported figures.

The numbers have changed substantially over the years. Edwin Oakes Jordan in *Epidemic Influenza: A Survey*, published by the American Medical Association in 1927, estimated the global total was 21.5 million. This remained the standard figure for decades, because so few had an interest in the pandemic. But historians have come to call Oakes's number "ludicrously low." As historians have taken more interest in the pandemic, they have revised Oakes's figures ever upward, sometimes significantly. While little is still known about places such as Russia and China, the most recent global estimate is fifty million; some think that figure may be an underestimate by as much as 100 percent.

Some countries, and even regions within countries, were hit much harder than others; mortality also differed based on age and gender. Indigenous people in Australia, New Zealand, and the United States suffered mortality rates as much as four times greater than the surrounding populations. In the remote native village of Wales in far northern Alaska, influenza was a virgin soil epidemic: 157 people died out of a total population of only 310. India, where approximately eighteen million died, had by far the highest death toll. Just as in other places, India's deaths from flu—mysteriously—were concentrated among young adults. This was quite different than previous flu epidemics and routine yearly outbreaks in which the elderly and the very young were disproportionally affected. In India women were hardest hit, because they took care of the sick. One result of both the age-specific mortality and the greater proportion of deaths among women was a marked lowering of the birth rate in India in subsequent years—as much as a 30 percent decline in 1919. There were fewer women, and many couples were no more.

The pandemic reached some of the most remote communities in the world. In the Pacific Islands the flu was devastating—mortality rates were higher in these islands than anywhere else. Almost no island lost less than 5 percent of its population. Western Samoa was the hardest hit: 22 percent of its population of about 38,000 died in a matter of weeks. If that happened today in the United States, seventy million would be dead. While the American naval administration was able to keep flu more or less out of American Samoa by strictly quarantining passengers on incoming ships and preventing mail boats from docking, such measures were never tried in Western Samoa. As a result, flu arrived aboard the New Zealand steamship *Talune*. Upon departure the ship had been given a clean bill of health, but in the week between its taking off from New Zealand and docking in Western Samoa flu became serious in New Zealand. No one warned Western Samoa or other ports of call. The islands learned about the pandemic from newspapers aboard the *Talune*, or from the devastating effects of the flu itself. Even though Western Samoa, like New Zealand, was part of the British Empire and the disease was well known all across the Pacific world, no one warned the islands of the unusually deadly nature of this particular flu outbreak. Within days, the island was overtaken. Ninety percent of the population was sick; social, administrative, and economic life ground to a halt.

The pandemic's virulence was blamed on the moral failings of Pacific islanders. The British agent on Tonga wrote: "The most discouraging feature of the outbreak was the apathy and indifference of the native chiefs to the suffering and distress of their people. . . . When conditions were at their worst . . . not a single Tongan was procurable for the most urgent work." These moral failings had political consequences: "Such incidents cause one to revise one's estimate of the Tongan character and show them incapable of deep feeling and unfitted for the high responsibilities of self-government." The 95 percent morbidity rate left few capable of vigorous action. Yet British observers blamed the islanders for the lackluster response to the epidemic while cheering their own efforts as heroic.

So appalling was the death rate in Western Samoa and so many were the questions left in its wake—principally, how could this have happened in an increasingly well-connected world where news traveled fast?—that in the summer of 1919 the British Colonial Office formed the Samoan Epidemic Commission to investigate why influenza was allowed to pass to Western Samoa and other islands when it was successfully kept out of neighboring American Samoa. One of the questions was "whether the introduction and extension of the said epidemic was caused by any negligence or default on the part of any persons in the service of the Crown, whether in respect of the Executive Government of New Zealand or in respect of the administration of the said Islands of Western Samoa."

The answer was yes. The commission determined that administrative bungling caused the failure to relay any information on the flu. Further, the commission found, the British administration in Western Samoa did not take the epidemic seriously enough; doctors assumed that their command of modern medicine would prevent the worst ravages of the disease. The failure to communicate was not limited to Western Samoa. The Colonial Office notified no one; the colonies themselves did a better job of telling their neighbors if they had flu. The dissemination of news was haphazard at best. Since flu was not a notifiable disease, news reached a given colony only when, for instance, Sierra Leone and the Gambia chose to notify neighboring Nigeria or someone read about it in the newspaper, or, worst of all, when the flu itself appeared.

That the pandemic was devastating is clear. The reason why is anything but. Pandemic influenza was not new, nor would the 1918 event be the last. Pandemics have been a regular feature of human history since the sixteenth century. Flu has been a yearly visitor for much longer. There had been a pandemic just a generation before in 1889–1890, and there would be later ones in 1957, 1968, and 2009. There will likely be another. But the 1918 pandemic was different.

Influenza is a virus—one with three types, of which influenza A is the most lethal and widespread. It is a zoonosis—a disease transmitted to humans from animals. The 1918 strain had not been seen before; it took until 2005 to even identify the virus as a strain of H1N1 (where H stands for hemagglutinin and N for neuraminidase; both are proteins) that had several distinguishing features. It struck young adults at a rate twenty times higher than during previous flu pandemics and the regular seasonal outbreaks, which generally had (and have) a far greater impact on the young and the old. Infection often led quickly to a deadly form of pneumonia. Mortality was much higher than in any other flu pandemic. Three separate waves, stacked one atop the other, left no time to recover or prepare.

Why all this was so still remains largely a mystery, its severity especially so. What is known from archival samples of the virus— which in 2005 allowed for a complete genomic sequencing of at least the fall 1918 virus—is that it is the ancestor of all four of the human and swine strains of what are called H1N1 and H2N2 lineages. But when it arrived in 1918 it was novel. It is possible that it originated in humans and then jumped to pigs. Yet not enough is known to say for sure, nor is it clear when it split into its human and porcine lineages. The genetic similarities between modern swine and human flu as well as the long-term association between influenza in pigs and people led flu researchers to conclude that pigs were the likely intermediary between the constantly circulating influenzas in animals and periodic pandemics in humans.

Until 1997. That year a virulent, deadly strain of avian influenza from Hong Kong, known as H5N1, jumped to humans directly. But so far H5N1 has been transmitted only from poultry to humans; human-to-human transmission has not yet definitively happened. It has become clearer and clearer that influenza A's largest reservoir is in fact avian—waterfowl, specifically. The discovery that avian influenza can pass directly to humans has upended previous models of flu transmission and alarmed virologists—who once thought this impossible—and public health officials. Added to influenza's ability to jump from animals to humans and back is that it changes rapidly and often (this is why we need a new flu vaccine more or less every autumn) via a process known as antigenic drift. Reassortment is a form of antigenic drift that occurs when different strains of the virus are mixed to produce a new strain; this is what happened, it seems, in 1918, 1957, and 1968. In the future it is possible that H5N1 will change in such a way that it becomes transmissible between humans, causing a new pandemic in a population of susceptible hosts.

Because flu is such a shape shifter, a group of prominent influenza researchers wrote in 2010, "Despite continuing progress in many areas, including enhanced human and animal surveillance and large-scale viral genomic screening, we are probably no better able today to anticipate and prevent the emergence of pandemic influenza than 5 centuries ago, as shown by the completely unexpected emergence of the 2009 novel H1N1 pandemic virus."

While we know a tremendous amount about the disease, there is much that still eludes us. That elusiveness, combined with influenza's power, is humbling. The 1918 pandemic arrived at a time when modern medicine had a newfound confidence in its ability to discover the causes of diseases and then offer cures. Yet before the development of vaccines in the 1940s and beyond, it was utterly defenseless against influenza.

But medical science did not know that. Beginning in the 1890s influenza was thought, erroneously, to be a bacterial infection— called Pfeiffer's bacillus after its discoverer, the German infectious disease specialist Johann Friedrich Pfeiffer. During the pandemic a raft of vaccines appeared, as did countless attempted remedies. None worked. Bacteriology was of no use. It was not until virology had matured enough that influenza was determined, in 1933, to be a virus. During the pandemic nothing could prevent it or cure it.

In the colonies modern medicine was no more effective than the frequently criticized "native" medicine it was supposed to replace. Colonial officials and expatriate doctors registered displeasure with the ineffectiveness of Western medicine, which strengthened local peoples' ties to traditional healers. In Bombay, this led to renewed interest in Ayurvedic and Unani medicine. In Sierra Leone, colonial authorities' handling of the pandemic prompted an editorial in the *Sierra Leone Weekly News* to opine, "The epidemic ought...to be made a distinct point of departure in the history of our country. It has been made ten times plainer...that our welfare lies in our standing up and doing things for ourselves." Not actually having effective treatment did not stop doctors from offering a wide array of "cures." The native commissioner in Belingwe, Southern Rhodesia, achieved "remarkable results" from a combination of mustard plaster, castor oil, brandy, and what he called "pneumonia mixture." Others used paraffin and sugar. Confident at first in these remedies, colonial administrators and doctors eventually admitted that Africans saw these "cures" for what they were: quackery. The Native Department reluctantly admitted that the progress doctors and clinics had made in convincing people to abandon indigenous medicine vanished as people "lost much of their confidence in the efficacy of European medicine." Africans associated the taking of European medicine with death and sickness. In parts of Southern Rhodesia, Africans kept outbreaks of the flu secret, fearing that sufferers would be sent to the dreaded lazaretto (isolation hospital) or be forced to take medicine many considered worse than the disease. This is not to suggest that African responses were effective, or that abandoning European medicine for Ayurvedic helped. It did not. No system was effective.

When influenza first appeared in Bloemfontein, South Africa, initial reactions were muted. The city considered itself so healthy that a local guidebook called it "the South African sanatorium." So confident was the city in its ability to ward off ill health that in early October, while flu was killing people in west Africa, the local newspaper wondered how dangerous "our friend the ordinary common or garden influenza" could be. They soon had an answer as bodies piled up and hospitals became overwhelmed. An elder of the Dutch Reformed Church said later in October, "It seemed to me that it was the end of mankind." The shock thrust the municipality into action—cinemas and schools were closed; local pharmacists were compelled to make their "flu mixtures" available to the public at no charge; black South Africans were conscripted as laborers to dig graves.

England, a country with one of the most robust public health infrastructures, mounted one of the weakest responses. Armed with a newfound faith in germ theory, physicians were convinced that they could tackle the disease and refused to accept that they had no real preventative or curative measures. Further, many medical professionals believed that fear fostered flu's progress, causing people to run about spreading the disease. Public health officials urged calm. This, combined with their overconfidence in modern medicine, led them to downplay the severity of the pandemic. Publications like the *British Medical Journal* counseled silence and inaction: one editorial said, "When epidemics occur, deaths always happen. Would it not be better if a little more prudence were shown in publishing such reports instead of banking up as many dark clouds as possible to upset our breakfasts?" An editorial in the *Manchester Guardian* echoed this sentiment: "Terror is a big ally of the influenza, and if the public state of mind can be steered out of the channel of fright a long, long step will have been taken to conquer the epidemic." Overreaction was frowned upon, especially in the face of war. As the *Times* remarked in December: "Never since the Black Death has such a plague swept over the face of the world; never, perhaps, has a plague been more stoically accepted."

On the advice of doctors, London's Local Government Board did little more than order that cinemas be well ventilated. Because of the strength of their faith in the germ theory, which was capable of lulling people into thinking cures and preventions were imminent, insufficient resources were directed toward mitigating some of the flu's effects. World War I had a profound impact—on morale, on the availability of doctors (so many were away), on the availability of resources generally. It proved tough to mobilize Britain to fight both a war abroad and a pandemic at home. Arthur Newsholme, chief medical officer of the Local Government Board, wrote:

> There are national circumstances in which the major duty is to "carry on," even when risk to life and health is involved. This duty has arisen as regards influenza. . . . It has arisen among munition workers and other workers engaged in work of national importance. . . . In each of the cases cited some lives might have been saved, spread of infection diminished, some suffering avoided, if the known sick could have been isolated from the healthy; if rigid exclusion of known sick and drastic increase of floor space for each person could have been enforced in factories, workplaces, barracks and ships; if overcrowding could have been regardlessly prohibited. But it was necessary to "carry on."

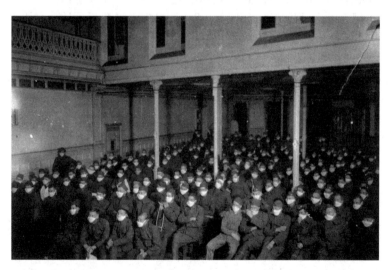

8. Fearing the flu, soldiers donned masks to watch a film in France during World War I.

Over the course of a few weeks in the fall of 1918, flu killed 250,000 people in England. Doctors and others distracted by war did not take the epidemic as seriously as they might have, but many people did recognize the magnitude of the crisis. As the *Times* put it: "So vast was the catastrophe and so ubiquitous its prevalence that our minds, surfeited with the horrors of war, refused to realize it. It came and went, a hurricane across the green fields of life, sweeping away our youth in hundreds of thousands and leaving behind it a toll of sickness and infirmity which will not be reckoned in this generation."

In the United States, initially, the Public Health Service published pamphlets that suggested the flu spreading across the country was in most ways no worse than the average annual flu. In the face of mounting cases, New York City's health commissioner continued throughout the first weeks of October 1918 to downplay the seriousness of the disease. Confident that the city could handle it, he cautioned citizens to remain calm; fear would only make things worse. In Italy, civil authorities forced the country's most influential newspaper, *Corriere della Sera*, to stop publishing the death toll as fear and anxiety mounted. These initially cavalier responses did give way to action in many places as municipalities realized the seriousness of the pandemic. Yet medicine was still ineffective.

Despite its failures, the appeal of modern medicine was scarcely diminished. The laboratory revolution had ushered in a new age; there was no turning back. Yet many physicians and public health experts were willing to admit their limitations. Thinking back on the pandemic in 1919, the bacteriologist Milton J. Rosenau wrote in the *Journal of the American Medical Association,* "If we have learned anything, it is that we are not quite sure what we know about the disease." This kind of admission was not uncommon, and at least in the United States it did not lead to despair; it pointed medical scientists toward opportunities.

The pandemic's effects are hard to gauge. Most historical work has focused on the pandemic itself, not what came after. Biomedical researchers, not historians, have taken the keenest interest. The appearance of H5N1 and the 2009 swine flu pandemic—which did not amount to the global nightmare that was predicted— sparked an extraordinary amount of research into the origins and implications of the 1918 pandemic. The pandemic has had a profound effect on twentieth- and twenty-first-century virology generally. But many historical questions remain. Some things do seem clear. For one, as a result of the disaster in the Pacific, as well as calls from New Zealand and South Africa to make flu a notifiable disease, there emerged a system of empire-wide disease surveillance and reporting. The system remained moribund until after World War II, but the pandemic did spawn an interest in a better system of international influenza surveillance—a system that is now considerably more robust.

But what of its cultural, economic, political, social, and demographic effects? From what little we do know, it seems to have had little impact in America. The pandemic has been all but forgotten. Its impact is barely detectable in memory or literature. Aside from the few books solely devoted to it, the pandemic rarely features in any substantial way in histories of the time. But could the same possibly be true in India, where nearly twenty million people died? Perhaps, but we don't know.

In many places in Africa—Southern Rhodesia, Nigeria, Zaire, and South Africa, for example—there arose a series of Pentecostal, or spirit, churches. The Aladura churches in Nigeria and the Kimbanguist Church in Zaire, for instance, formed when prophets, directed by God, appeared to save their people from the ravages of the flu. Pentecostal churches that emerged in Southern Rhodesia in the immediate aftermath of the flu's arrival remained long after the pandemic was gone.

In Bloemfontein, South Africa, the pandemic sparked a number of immediate changes in public health laws and invigorated a move toward poor relief as the city was forced to face the fact that it was not as healthy or as slum-free as it imagined. "The citizens were...shocked at the revelation of slums and degradation disclosed by the 'Flu'" announced the city's town clerk and treasurer. One of the city's newspapers, the *Friend*, wrote, "The immediate result has been a stimulating of the public conscience in the direction of long-delayed social reforms. Schemes are now under consideration which were regarded yesterday as the dreams of impracticable visionaries, and to-day are demanded as urgent necessities." Reform had been tossed about before, but it took the pandemic to shock the city into action. As the mayor told the Influenza Epidemic Commission, "Bloemfontein had long had such a scheme in contemplation, but the experience in the epidemic had hastened matters and stimulated public opinion, which was now ripe for these reforms." For now, one can only wonder if the pandemic caused similar reforms elsewhere, to say nothing of its possible effects on other aspects of life.

The 1918 influenza pandemic was an event. Unlike malaria and tuberculosis—the perpetual pandemics—influenza comes and goes. In this way it is more like smallpox or plague. Of course those two diseases are no longer major global threats. Influenza is. When H5N1 appeared in humans in 1997 and the novel strain of H1N1 turned up in 2009, the world was reminded of the possibility of another 1918. It has not happened yet. We do not know when it will. We are rather like the English in the seventeenth century. They knew that plague was out there, lurking, ready to strike, and they were more or less resigned to its return. They did not know when or why it would come back; they did, mostly, know how: by ship from abroad. Protecting themselves, once they knew it was coming, by keeping plague out was the only thing that had any potential of warding off an epidemic. We have vaccines now, a robust global monitoring system, and in some places a well-run public health infrastructure. Yet we are still like our seventeenth-century counterparts anxiously watching the shore.

Further, in the event of a deadly pandemic many of the same things that keep tuberculosis and malaria alive and well in the resource-poor parts of the world—among other things lack of public health infrastructure, inadequate access to preventive medicine, compromised immune systems, and rampant co-infections—will ensure that, just as in 1918, any future influenza pandemic will have wildly divergent effects.

While we are now sufficiently aware of the challenges of tackling the flu, and unlike in 1918 most virologists and public health officials do not possess an unhealthy amount of confidence, it can be hard to muster concern. For many, flu is simply synonymous with a cold. Both the 1976 swine flu and 2009's H1N1 pandemic amounted to much less than many public health officials predicted they would be. These things all can add up to a generally lackadaisical outlook when it comes to general concern about the possibility of a deadly pandemic. This is a mistake.

Chapter 7
HIV/AIDS

The arrival of HIV/AIDS was the end of the age of hubris. Any bluster about the death of infectious disease by the hand of biomedicine or hope of living in a world free of pestilence disappeared as it became clear that HIV/AIDS was a new infectious disease thriving in a world thought to be on the verge of being free of such menaces.

HIV/AIDS had been percolating in central Africa since the early twentieth century, but it appeared in its now recognizable form in the spring of 1981, when doctors in Los Angeles and New York City began noticing a strange uptick in rare diseases like pneumocystis carinii pneumonia (a fungal infection to which immunocompromised individuals are susceptible) and Kaposi's sarcoma (a rare form of cancer, mostly found in the aged). Even stranger was that they clustered in sexually active gay men. Then, over the next year or so, other groups, including hemophiliacs and intravenous drug users, became similarly afflicted. People from Haiti, too, seemed to be struck down. A Belgian doctor, Peter Piot, keeping up with the news from Centers for Disease Control, recognized similarities between what he was reading about in the United States and what he was seeing in his clinic in Antwerp—a clinic frequented by African immigrants. More and more reports from other parts of the world began popping up of unexplained cases of Kaposi's sarcoma and an assortment of immune disorders.

What linked these groups? Why were they all suffering from a host of diseases that were both rare and generally able to be fought off by a healthy immune system? The biomedical community snapped to attention. Initially (and unfortunately), the CDC labeled it GRID (gay-related immunodeficiency disease). In the summer of 1982 it was given its formal and lasting name: AIDS (acquired immune deficiency syndrome). Not long after, in 1983 and 1984, respectively, the Pasteur Institute in France and the National Cancer Institute in the United States identified the virus. Each called it something different; each claimed credit for the sole discovery. But soon the medical community settled on a name: human immunodeficiency virus.

HIV/AIDS has now killed nearly thirty million and infected nearly seventy-five million people worldwide. Tens of thousands of new cases appear each year. No part of the inhabited globe has been untouched by HIV/AIDS. But not everywhere is affected equally: well more than a third of all cases and deaths have occurred in southern Africa. In some places, like the Middle East, Latin America, Japan, and parts of Europe, HIV/AIDS affects mostly socially marginalized portions of the population; in central, eastern, and southern Africa it is a problem of the general population. In 2004, data from prenatal clinics in Swaziland revealed a prevalence rate of 42.6 percent.

When considered alongside the agents responsible for the causes of other diseases, the discovery of HIV only two years after AIDS first came to medical attention is remarkable—it took millennia to understand what caused plague. Decades of advances in molecular biology, immunology, and virology saw to that. The rapid identification of the virus and the seemingly limitless US federal government spending on medical research (the United States spent far more than any other country on AIDS research) led to hasty predictions of a vaccine and for a time bolstered modern medicine's confidence in its own powers.

But the optimism did not last. Identifying the virus was not enough. HIV turned out to be a complex retrovirus with several different identities. There are actually two viruses: HIV-1 and HIV-2. HIV-1 is more prevalent; HIV-2 is largely confined to West Africa and is much slower moving and harder to transmit. HIV-1 is broken down into groups (M, N, O) and then further into eleven genetically distinct subtypes (A–K). Group M (the main group) is the one responsible for the pandemic, as it causes 99 percent of cases. Subtypes A, C, and D make up the vast majority of cases, about 84 percent. Subtype C accounts for most cases in southern Africa, India, and China—and thus for a huge proportion of the world's HIV.

HIV 1 and 2 are both zoonoses (diseases originating in animals that now infect humans), and each of the different types of HIV is an instance of separate transmissions from chimpanzees (HIV-1) or sooty mangabeys (HIV-2). The greatest genetic diversity of HIV is in central Africa. All group M subtypes are found there, as are many recombinant forms in which the virus's genetic makeup is different still. Such genetic diversity means this is the region where HIV has been developing the longest and is thus the origin point for the pandemic. The virus passed from chimpanzee to human sometime around the turn of the twentieth century when, more than likely, infected chimpanzee blood entered the body of a hunter through a cut or open sore. By about 1920 HIV had made its way to the area around Léopoldville (since 1966 Kinshasa). From there it made its way across Africa along ever developing transportation networks. Its speed accelerated in various places and times: colonial era medical campaigns against sleeping sickness, yaws, and syphilis frequently reused needles, thus allowing the virus to be transmitted quickly to large numbers of people. Passing HIV to female prostitutes by treating them for syphilis with non-sterile needles was an especially effective way of getting HIV into the general population in the 1950s and 1960s. Once enough prostitutes were infected, HIV spread, especially in the dramatically changing environment of Léopoldville in the

1960s—mass migration to the city, high unemployment, and an explosion in prostitution. From there HIV moved on to Haiti as the many Haitians employed by various United Nations agencies like UNESCO migrated back and forth between the two countries. It then spread to the rest of the world.

HIV is very difficult to control. For one, because it is a lentivirus, it develops very slowly during a lengthy incubation. The genetic material of all life, including most viruses, is DNA. But HIV is a retrovirus, which means that HIV's genetic material is found in RNA (ribonucleic acid). When HIV invades a cell, it converts itself to DNA and then makes copies of its genetic material, via an enzyme called reverse transcriptase, as RNA. During the conversion, HIV makes many, many mistakes in copying itself, and the virus mutates. Because HIV changes so rapidly and so unpredictably, making a vaccine is difficult—so far it has proven impossible. HIV makes its way into the body via infected fluids—blood and semen are the most effective. Heterosexual transmission is most common. However, mother-to-child transmission, non-sterile needles used for intravenous drugs, and men having sex with men are all critically important routes by which the virus travels. Once in the body, HIV attacks the immune system's CD4 cells. Especially important is that HIV targets two types of CD4 cells essential for fighting infections: the T helper cells, which are the body's main defense against foreign bodies and infections, and the macrophages, which seize foreign bodies and allow the immune system to recognize these invaders. Once infected, seroconversion—the process by which HIV antibodies develop in the body and the virus becomes detectable—occurs. The strength of the infection is measured by viral load; a person is most infectious shortly after infection.

HIV progresses through four stages based on the CD4 count—a healthy individual's CD4 count is more than 1,000 cells per cubic millimeter of blood. At stage 1 the CD4 count is usually greater than 500, and the individual is asymptomatic. Once at stage 2

CD4 has dropped to between 350 and 499, and symptoms like weight loss and fungal infections may appear. In stage 3 CD4 count has dropped below 350. The individual is severely immunocompromised and susceptible to many opportunistic infections. Full-blown AIDS, when the CD4 count is below 200, is stage 4. As a virus, HIV's main features are its stunning complexity and insidious ability to disable the very system designed to repel it.

Added to all this are the political and social factors that determine its control. They involve sexual behavior, gender, poverty, and access to medicine, as well as political will—or lack thereof. Yet because HIV/AIDS arrived at a time of scientific triumphalism, a time when the biomedical community felt powerfully that a biomedical solution was best and was imminent, there has always been a tension between the social and medical aspects of dealing with pandemic. Very broadly speaking, the biomedical response has been nothing short of breathtaking. An entirely new scientific industry has been created. Breakthroughs in understanding were rapid and frequent. As a result, the disease went from a nearly always fatal, virtually untreatable affliction to a manageable chronic disease in less than a generation.

But the biomedical breakthroughs have not always been in sync with life outside the lab. HIV/AIDS is now treatable, but access to drugs is uneven, and new infections continue to demonstrate that prevention efforts have been only partly successful. From the very beginning of the pandemic the response has been fraught with many, many challenges. In the United States, for example, where the disease has primarily been associated with sexually active gay men and intravenous drug users, panic, fear, and moral opprobrium were common reactions. Conservative senators such as Jesse Helms blamed gay men: AIDS was retribution for sinful behavior. Needle exchange programs, which have a demonstrable public health benefit, have always been controversial, thought by many to promote illegal drug use. Many perceived government agencies like the Food and Drug Administration to be slow and ineffective at approving new drugs in a timely manner. As a result, a powerful and effective AIDS activist movement, exemplified by ACT UP, emerged to challenge bureaucratic dithering.

Safe-sex programs ran into opposition from those who considered abstinence the best way to avoid HIV/AIDS; condom use was also slow to take hold among men who visited prostitutes, and some men simply refused to use them at all; and as the epidemic began to level off in the United States, the use of condoms diminished. Outside the United States the national responses to the pandemic have been so varied that generalization is not possible. Some countries were passive, while others took a more active approach. Cuba instituted strict isolation of those who were HIV positive and mandated testing for the entire country. In Africa, Uganda confronted the epidemic head-on right from the start, advocating for and promoting a campaign aimed at reducing the number of sexual partners individuals had. Other countries, such as Zimbabwe, denied even having the disease within its borders.

If measured in dollars spent, papers published, careers launched, and breakthroughs achieved, the biomedical response to the pandemic was extraordinary. The political and social responses were less so. Writing in *The Lancet* in 2008, several prominent physicians from the pandemic's early years claimed that the global response "was for the most part delayed, grossly insufficient, fragmented, and inconsistent."

One area of striking neglect was Africa, which was both the origin point and the epicenter of the pandemic. The reasons are varied and complex and are both indigenous and endogenous. Most considered AIDS to be a gay disease, and thus considerable stigma was attached to it. There were exceptions: Uganda and Senegal publicly confronted AIDS, admitted it was present, and worked to confine their epidemics by not stigmatizing the ill. In South Africa, denialism reached a peak in the mid-1990s when President

Thabo Mbeki and his minister of health argued, following the American denialist Peter Duesberg, that HIV did not cause AIDS and thus newly emerging and effective drugs would be useless.

The WHO was slow to take notice. Four years into the pandemic, Halfdan Mahler, the director general, still did not consider HIV/AIDS a priority. He stated, "AIDS is not spreading like a bush fire in Africa. It is malaria and other diseases that are killing millions of children every day." Further, the pandemic looked much different in Africa. In the United States and much of Europe, where the vast majority of research was being conducted, the disease most affected gay men and intravenous drug users. Biomedical research and policy largely focused on the disease's profile in the countries where the research was taking place. Heterosexual transmission was initially rare and not considered a driver of the epidemic. Relief set in among some in the United States as it became clear that AIDS was largely confined to "high risk" groups; the tidal wave of heterosexual AIDS many feared never came.

The consequences for Africa were great. The dismissal of heterosexual transmission as unimportant in the United States meant that the burgeoning heterosexual pandemic erupting in Africa—so effectively documented by the pathbreaking work of Project SIDA in Congo—was initially ignored. This meant too that the burden of HIV in women went unexamined. By the time the WHO started its Special Programme on AIDS (soon renamed the Global Programme on AIDS; GPA) in 1987, the pandemic had been silently spreading more or less unabated.

Once the GPA was created and Jonathan Mann (who had been running Project SIDA in Congo and who would go on to become a legend in the HIV/AIDS world) hired to run it, global AIDS received unprecedented attention; donations to WHO skyrocketed. The GPA had success in working with Uganda and Thailand to dramatically reduce transmission, and Mann successfully turned to nongovernmental organizations for help. The GPA also made HIV/AIDS a human rights issue in an effort to reduce stigma and ensure that individuals would not suffer discrimination and persecution. For a short time, the WHO attempted to think of TB and HIV in unison, recognizing that HIV was having and would continue to have a considerable impact on TB. The GPA operated more or less autonomously—which led in part to its downfall—and was WHO's largest and best funded program. When Mahler and Mann addressed the UN General Assembly in the fall of 1987, it was the first time in history that a disease appeared on the assembly's agenda. WHO was the leader in tackling global AIDS.

But HIV/AIDS's time in the spotlight was short-lived. Mann resigned in 1990, after repeatedly clashing with the director general, Hiroshi Nakajima. The GPA lost momentum. Not long after, the WHO closed the GPA. AIDS work moved to a new agency, UNAIDS, in an effort to consolidate activities in one place. In the transitional years from the end of Mann's tenure to UNAIDS reaching operational capacity—albeit far below that of the GPA—global HIV/AIDS was left leaderless and adrift.

Not many people were paying attention anyway. So focused were they on the domestic epidemic that both the AIDS activist movement in the United States and the US government itself virtually ignored AIDS in the developing world. And, tragically, these were the very same years that the pandemic began to increase exponentially in Africa. While AIDS briefly occupied the global stage during the early years of the GPA, attention flagged, and by the early 1990s, even though the majority of cases were in the developing world, it only received 6 percent of global spending on HIV prevention. Due to profound neglect and craven political calculation much valuable ground was lost in the 1990s. When UNAIDS published its book-length history of the global response to the pandemic, it pulled no punches: during the decade and a half after the first case appeared, they wrote, "the world's leaders, in all sectors of society, had displayed a staggering indifference to the growing challenge of this new epidemic."

Beyond simple neglect, overall aid to developing countries declined dramatically in the 1980s and into the 1990s. UN agencies like the WHO suffered when donor nations like the United States during the Reagan years refused to pay dues (though for a time the GPA was an exception, as it received earmarked funds). Neoliberal economic policies forced countries to accept austerity in order to pay down their large burdens of debt. HIV/AIDS began to have an enormous effect on economies at the same time as the effects of structural adjustment programs continued to sap countries' already meager reserves just when they needed resources the most. The effects were staggering. One result, among others, was that funding for healthcare plummeted; many African countries introduced user fees—fees few patients were able to pay.

During these years, too, the World Bank gained in importance while the WHO declined. Beginning in 1987, the same year GPA opened, the bank began funding more and more health programs based on neoliberal principles which meant, among other things, that health interventions would be evaluated based on analysis of cost-effectiveness; it also meant that many countries' public health budgets sharply declined. As the bank took on a larger and larger role in funding health programs, it naturally gained more and more influence over what those programs looked like. One of the most powerful effects was coming to see disease interventions in terms of cost-effectiveness. This new way of prioritizing programs made its debut in the World Bank's 1993 *World Development Report: Investing in Health*, which signaled to the world, according to an editorial in *The Lancet*, that a shift had occurred "in leadership in international health from the World Health Organization to the World Bank." The bank sought to identify (and the WHO followed along) which diseases had the most deleterious effects on the economy—measured in what are called

DALYs (disability-adjusted life years)—while also being relatively inexpensive to treat. By any measure, according to those calculating things in such terms, treating AIDS was not cost-effective. Because the newly emerging class of antiretroviral drugs was expensive, they were not cost-effective in low income countries. Some HIV prevention efforts, such as condoms, were considered cost-effective, but they were very hard to implement.

Thus developing countries were in a strange, perhaps ironic, position: just as the holy grail of the global north's pursuit of a technological fix was in sight—highly active antiretroviral therapy (HAART)—the global south was told by the north it could not have it; it costs too much. It would be more cost-effective to work on preventing HIV instead. The very same economic imperatives that led the United States to fixate on a biomedical solution to the neglect of social interventions were now preventing an effective biomedical intervention from reaching those most in need.

The 1990s was a decade of neglect and lost opportunity. The global political response to HIV/AIDS in the 1990s was inadequate. The same cannot be said of biomedicine. In 1995 and 1996 two new classes of antiretroviral drugs had been discovered, tested, and released: the first were protease inhibitors—first saquinavir, and then the non-nucleoside reverse transcriptase inhibitors, beginning with nevirapine. At the eleventh International AIDS Conference in Vancouver researchers announced that when drugs from these two different classes were used in a triple combination, the virus could be suppressed and the patient's immune systems restored.

A disease that had been a death sentence was no longer fatal. One of these drugs, nevirapine, not only helped those with HIV; it could also prevent its transmission to babies. Mother-to-infant transmission had been (and still is) a challenging problem, but giving a dose of nevirapine to the mother just before birth and the baby just after has a dramatic effect on this route of transmission.

Where access has been greatest, mother-to-child transition rates have dropped significantly. Tragically, nevirapine was kept out of South Africa's antenatal clinics until 2002—when the Constitutional Court intervened to make them available—because of Thabo Mbeki's belief that HIV did not cause AIDS.

With the advent of these new drugs it was possible that AIDS could become a chronic manageable disease, thus altering the course of the pandemic. But they were expensive—prohibitively so for many people. They cost $10,000 to $15,000 per year and needed to be taken for life. Insuring access would be critical. Meanwhile, in the United States mortality from AIDS-related causes began dropping in the late 1990s—between 1996 and 1997 alone it fell 46 percent. The domestic epidemic became less urgent, and the international pandemic continued to be virtually ignored.

Added to this were arguments from some in global health leadership that treating AIDS in the developing world was neither cost-effective nor feasible for lack of infrastructure. Two articles in *The Lancet* made this claim. One claimed that "data on the cost-effectiveness of HIV prevention in sub-Saharan Africa and on highly active antiretroviral therapy indicate that prevention is at least 28 times more cost-effective than HAART." The other argued: "The most cost-effective interventions are for prevention of HIV/AIDS and treatment of tuberculosis, while HAART for adults, and home based care organized from health facilities, are the least cost-effective." Treatment and prevention were deemed mutually exclusive. In the world in which many operated, these kinds of stark choices were thought to be necessary. Further, the head of USAID told the US House of Representatives, Africans were generally incapable of taking such drugs even if they were available, because, among other reasons, Africans do not wear watches; their way of rendering time is different, and thus they would not be able to adhere to a treatment schedule.

But then a tectonic shift occurred. Beginning around the turn of the millennium there emerged a new way of seeing the pandemic. Global health became a priority for the United States government and major philanthropies such as the Bill and Melinda Gates Foundation. For example, in 2000 the United States funded antiretroviral therapy (ART) for no more than a few hundred patients around the world; by September 2009 the State Department claimed that the United States was providing ART for 2.5 million people.

What explains this shift in funding and interest? Drug policy and cost. For much of the 1990s second-line drugs for drug-resistant tuberculosis and ART were extraordinarily expensive. Many in global health accepted this as fixed costs rather than human constructions. In the early 1980s, ACT UP pioneered AIDS activism centered on access to treatment. In the late 1990s a new generation of activists emerged in South Africa and demanded access to antiretrovirals and answers to a series of hard questions: What does it mean to say the drugs cost too much? Who decides? Who sets prices? To activists the answer was that if high prices were set by people, then they could also be lowered. And if the cost of drugs dropped, then arguments about them not being cost-effective would disappear.

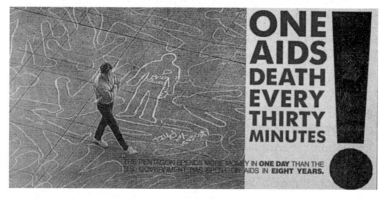

ONE AIDS DEATH EVERY THIRTY MINUTES

THE PENTAGON SPENDS MORE MONEY IN **ONE DAY** THAN THE U.S. GOVERNMENT HAS SPENT ON AIDS IN **EIGHT YEARS.**

9. **During the 1980s and 1990s, ACT UP drew attention to what many considered the lackluster US response to the AIDS epidemic.**

Things began to happen on many fronts. Research began appearing to counter the claims of non-adherence and suggestions that prevention and treatment were mutually exclusive ends. Two studies of the limited role out of HAART appeared in 2001—one coming out of Haiti and the other out of Khayelitsha, outside Cape Town—that demonstrated people stayed on treatment. In the Cape Town study scientists learned even more: with the increase in availability of treatment, more and more people sought testing. That is, when people saw that there was effective treatment, more and more sought out AIDS services. As more people knew their status, and more began to receive treatment, transmission declined.

Clearly, HAART could work in resource-poor settings. But drugs still cost a tremendous amount. In India and Brazil, drug manufacturers began to produce cheaper generic versions of commercial ARVs. But in the rest of the world patents prevented drugs from being made in generic forms, and pharmaceutical companies, aided by the United States and the World Trade Organization, worked to keep generics out of global circulation. In 1997 South Africa attempted to challenge this by passing the Medicines Act, which stipulated that in the case of a public health emergency such as AIDS the country was allowed to both produce and import generic versions of drugs that were still patent-protected.

Claiming that the law violated their intellectual property rights, in 1998 thirty-nine drug companies reacted by filing suit in South African court. Activists, especially the Treatment Action Campaign, argued that the costs of the drugs were far out of proportion to their research and development outlay, to say nothing of the humanitarian argument for making them available.

The Clinton administration supported the drug makers, going so far as to put South Africa on a "watch list"—the precursor to sanctions—citing the possibility that the Medicines Act would "abrogate patent rights." When Vice President Al Gore announced

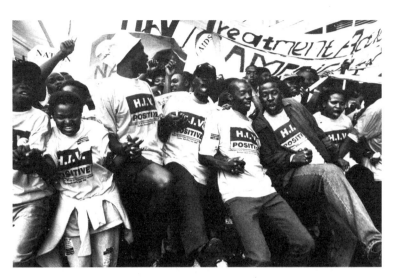

10. **Treatment Action Campaign protestors demand free access to life-saving drugs in the streets of Durban, South Africa, in July 2000. This powerful image contradicts the popular perception of the disease and helpless "African" AIDS victims.**

his candidacy for the presidency, protestors suddenly appeared behind him with banners that read "Gore's greed kills! AIDS drugs for Africa!" Protests broke out elsewhere, and within three months the US government reversed course: the United States would not pressure any country into purchasing only brand names and would allow importation of generics. By April 2001 all thirty-nine drug companies had dropped their suits. The door was now open for cheap generics to fill the gap in treatment.

Alongside the change in drug policy came a massive increase in funding. And one of the biggest funders—as well as one of the biggest surprises—was the President's Emergency Plan for AIDS Relief (PEPFAR), announced on January 28, 2003, during President George W. Bush's State of the Union Address. Bush said:

> AIDS can be prevented. Antiretroviral drugs can extend life many years.... Seldom has history offered a greater opportunity to do so

much for so many.... To meet a severe and urgent crisis abroad, tonight I propose the Emergency Plan for AIDS Relief—a work of mercy beyond all current international efforts to help the people of Africa.... I ask the Congress to commit $15 billion over the next five years, including nearly $10 billion in new money, to turn the tide against AIDS in the most afflicted nations of Africa and the Caribbean.

PEPFAR aimed to quickly scale up access to ARTs, modeled in part after work being done in Uganda.

By the middle of the first decade of the new century a combination of factors changed the face of AIDS funding and treatment: lower drug prices, growing evidence of the efficacy of treatment in resource-poor settings, grassroots activism, and new funding sources such as PEPFAR. However, access remains uneven, and new infections mean access will have to expand if the pandemic is to be stopped. Funding sources are fickle. Stigma and lack of understanding still hinder progress. Even in the United States, where activism and access has arguably been the greatest, African American men and women in places like Washington, DC, have rates far exceeding those of the white population—75 percent of new cases in 2013 were among the black population; likewise, 75 percent of those living with HIV/AIDS are black. During an outbreak of HIV among intravenous drug users in rural Indiana in 2015, it became clear that stigma was still a major problem when some addicts refused to get tested, as they feared being labeled as gay if they were seen coming and going from a local clinic; many did not know treatment was available or know the consequences of sharing used needles.

HIV/AIDS changed global health in fundamental ways: it spawned a vibrant and essential activist movement that changed the ways in which drugs are priced and accessed and also insisted on the link between health and human rights. The pandemic also made it clear that we will never live in a world free of disease.

It has also reminded us that we live in a world of starkly different opportunity and access—the fact that the overwhelming amount of HIV/AIDS is in the developing world should make this very clear. As with the other pandemic diseases, the global burden of HIV/AIDS rests on those least able to combat it.

Epilogue

What are we to do with this history? Does all this past experience, all this history, inform the present? Yes and no. In spring 2015 the WHO released a statement admitting its lackluster response to the Ebola pandemic and calling attention to a number of "lessons learned." It was a striking document. It was striking that in 2015 among the lessons learned were such things as the "lessons of community and culture." That it took Ebola to show the value of local people and their knowledge is surprising. The WHO "learned the importance of capacity"—which means the WHO learned that the world did not have the capacity to handle epidemics. The WHO was "reminded that market-based systems do not deliver commodities for neglected diseases." Why did it take Ebola to relearn that important fact? The WHO also learned that gains in such things as malaria control or women surviving childbirth can be reversed when "built on fragile health systems." Is it truly possible that this lesson had not been learned before 2015?

I am not interested in indicting the WHO—it is in this instance an easy target—and it is commendable that the leadership is admitting mistakes. But the WHO is, for better or worse, representative of a way of seeing things in the world of global health, and the leadership's statement on lessons learned allows me to make a point: every single lesson it learned (or in one instance relearned) could have been gleaned from a look at the past. These lessons are not new; the history of epidemics and pandemics has been teaching them for centuries. That there seems to be no historical consciousness is frustrating, but not just because I am a historian. It is frustrating because it is wasteful and inefficient. It is also arrogant and naive—a lethal combination. It is naive to think that by simply learning lessons the future will be different and arrogant to suppose that those proffering the mea culpas are the enlightened ones finally seeing the mistakes of the past. The WHO and others must ask: What are the origins of the mistakes themselves? That they were made is important, but the reason why might be more so.

Pandemics are not going away. There are no doubt more to come. A pandemic might come from an old and familiar foe such as influenza or might emerge from a new source—a zoonosis that has made its way into humans, perhaps. How will the world confront pandemics in the future? It is very likely that patterns established long ago will reemerge. But how will new challenges, like global climate change, affect future pandemics and our ability to respond? It is very likely that as the climate warms, disease-carrying mosquitoes, for example, will inhabit new places. Take the Zika virus. Carried by the *Aedes aegypti* mosquito—commonly referred to as the yellow fever mosquito—Zika exploded in early 2016 in Latin America and the Caribbean as temperatures set record highs and *Aedes aegypti* found suitable habitat. It is possible that as temperatures rise elsewhere, Zika will find a home further north. Rising water temperatures might provide more habitat for cholera. And as more and more research suggests a connection between the periodic rise in temperatures in central Asia and the arrival of plague in Europe in the late medieval period, we would do well to pay more attention to other instances of the historic connections between climate change and disease.

In the future, will nongovernmental organizations like Doctors Without Borders—the group that so heroically and tirelessly responded to Ebola while the world watched—be relied on as first responders? Or will the WHO regain some of its lost stature? One thing is clear: in the face of a serious pandemic much of the developing world's public health infrastructure will be woefully overburdened. One sure way to ease the suffering that will be encountered in any future pandemic is to invest in building a robust public health infrastructure anywhere one is lacking. The effects of pandemic and epidemic diseases have been and are going to be far worse in the places least able to respond. Although this might seem to be simple common sense, it is clear from the "lessons learned" by the WHO in the wake of the Ebola epidemic that it is still routinely forgotten.

Epilogue

References

Introduction

For the pandemic criteria see David M. Morens, Gregory K. Folkers, and Anthony S. Fauci, "What Is a Pandemic?," *Journal of Infectious Diseases* 200, no. 7 (2009): 1019–20.

Sanjoy Bhattacharya has written very effectively about the uses of history in contemporary discussions of epidemic disease: "International Health and the Limits of Its Global Influence: Bhutan and the Worldwide Smallpox Eradication Programme," *Medical History* 57, no. 4 (2013): 486.

Chapter 1: Plague

The quotes on the experience of the first plague pandemic are from Lester K. Little, "Life and Afterlife of the First Plague Pandemic," in *Plague and the End of Antiquity: The Pandemic of 541–570*, ed. Lester K. Little (Cambridge, UK: Cambridge University Press, 2007), 9.

For needing to employ such disciplines as zoology, archaeology, and molecular biology see Michael McCormick, "Rats, Communications, and Plague: Toward an Ecological History," *Journal of Interdisciplinary History* 34, no. 1 (2003): 25.

On the first plague pandemic in Britain see J. R. Maddicott, "Plague in Seventh Century England," *Past and Present* 156 (1997): 50.

The quotes from Ralph of Shrewsbury, the Paris masters, the *Decameron*, and the "French observer" are all from the essential volume *The Black Death*, trans. and ed. Rosemary Horrox (Manchester, UK: Manchester University Press, 1994), 112, 163, 26–27.

On Venice and Florence see Ann G. Carmichael, "Plague Legislation in the Italian Renaissance," *Bulletin of the History of Medicine* 57, no. 4 (1983): 511.

The details on labor shortages in England and Italy are from, respectively, John Hatcher, "England in the Aftermath of the Black Death," *Past and Present* 144 (1994): 3–35, and David Herlihy, *The Black Death and the Transformation of the West*, ed. Samuel K. Cohn, Jr. (Cambridge, MA: Harvard University Press, 1997); see 48–49 for Italian quotes. John de Wodhull is quoted in the manorial account of the royal manor of Drakelow in Cheshire, England, for 1349–1350. This is document 94 in Horrox, *Black Death*, quote on 283.

The Ibn al-Khatib quote is from John Aberth, *The First Horseman: Disease in Human History* (Upper Saddle River, NJ: Pearson, 2007).

Richard Leake and Stephen Bradwell are quoted in Paul Slack, *The Impact of Plague in Tudor and Stuart England* (Oxford: Clarendon, 1985), 39, 27.

The values quote is found in Vivian Nutton, "The Seeds of Disease: An Explanation of Contagion and Infection From the Greeks to the Renaissance," *Medical History* 27, no. 1 (1983): 31–32.

On earlier plagues not being *the* plague see Samuel K. Cohn, "The Black Death: End of a Paradigm," *American Historical Review* 107, no. 3 (2002): 737.

The president of the London Epidemiological Society is quoted in Mark Harrison, *Contagion: How Commerce Has Spread Disease* (New Haven, CT: Yale University Press, 2012), 185.

The *Mahratta* quote and the quote from the sanitary engineer are both in David Arnold, *Colonizing the Body: State Medicine and Epidemic Disease in Nineteenth-Century India* (Cambridge, UK: Cambridge University Press, 1993), 212, 232.

Chapter 2: Smallpox

The quote from Ho Chung is in Donald R. Hopkins, *The Greatest Killer: Smallpox in History* (Chicago: University Of Chicago Press, 2002), 104.

The quote from the Florentine Codex is found in John Mack Farther and Robert V. Hine, *The American West: A New Interpretive History* (New Haven, CT: Yale University Press, 2000), 22–23.

The quotes from the English colonists William Bradford and Thomas Hariot are from David S. Jones, *Rationalizing Epidemics: The Meanings and Uses of American Indian Mortality since 1600* (Cambridge, MA: Harvard University Press, 2004), 37, 26.

The concept of the Great Southeastern Smallpox Epidemic comes from Paul Kelton, *Epidemics and Enslavement: Biological Catastrophe in the Native Southeast, 1492–1715* (Lincoln: University of Nebraska Press, 2007).

For the Huron calling the French the "greatest sorcerers on earth" see Reuben Gold Thwaites, ed., *The Jesuit Relations: Travels and Explorations of the Jesuit Missionaries in New France, 1610–1791*, vol. 19, *Quebec and Hurons: 1640* (Cleveland: Burrows,, 1899), 91; this edition is a computerized transcription by Tomasz Mentrak, last updated April 14, 2011, available at http://puffin.creighton.edu/jesuit/relations/relations_19.html.

Truteau is quoted in Colin Calloway, *One Vast Winter Count: The Native American West before Lewis and Clark* (Lincoln: University of Nebraska Press, 2003), 419.

The Lewis and Clark quote is found in the online edition of *The Journals of Lewis and Clark Expedition*, based on the edition of the journals by Gary E. Moulton, available at http://lewisandclarkjournals.unl.edu/index.html.

Chapter 3: Malaria

The entomologist in Panama and *Mosquito Control in Panama* are quoted in Paul S. Sutter, "Nature's Agents or Agents of Empire?" *Isis* 98, no. 4 (2007): 743, 744.

Collins is quoted in Kenneth F. Kiple and Kriemhild Coneè Ornelas, "Race, War, and Tropical Medicine in the Eighteenth-Century Caribbean," in *Warm Climates and Western Medicine: The Emergence of Tropical Medicine, 1500–1900*, ed. David Arnold (Amsterdam: Rodopi, 1996), 73.

James Lind is quoted in E. C. Spary, "Health and Medicine in the Enlightenment," in *The Oxford Handbook of the History of Medicine*, ed. Mark Jackson (Oxford: Oxford University Press, 2011), 89.

Patrick Manson is quoted in Michael Worboys, "Germs, Malaria and the Invention of Mansonian Tropical Medicine: From 'Diseases in the Tropics' to 'Tropical Diseases,'" in Arnold, *Warm Climates and Western Medicine*, 194.

Bentley and Christophers are quoted in Ira Klein, "Malaria and Mortality in Bengal, 1840–1921," *Indian Economic and Social History Review* 9, no. 2 (1972): 142.

The Brazilian newspaper quote is in Randall M. Packard, *The Making of a Tropical Disease: A Short History of Malaria* (Baltimore: Johns Hopkins University Press, 2007), 96.

Paul Russell is quoted in Nancy Leys Stepan, *Eradication: Ridding the World of Diseases Forever?* (Ithaca, NY: Cornell University Press, 2011), 155.

McDermott is quoted in Walsh McDermott, "Environmental Factors Bearing on Medical Education in the Developing Countries," *Academic Medicine* 41, no. 9 (1966): S138.

The Cockburn quote is from T. Aidan Cockburn, "Eradication of Infectious Disease," *Science* 133, no. 3458 (April 7, 1961): 1058.

Chapter 4: Cholera

The Hamlin quote is in Christopher Hamlin, *Cholera: The Biography* (New York: Oxford University Press, 2009), 56.

For the quote from the French writer see Vijay Prashad, "Native Dirt/ Imperial Ordure: The Cholera of 1832 and the Morbid Resolutions of Modernity," *Journal of Historical Sociology* 7, no. 3 (1994): 247.

The quotes from the *Quarterly Review*, the *Medico-Chirurgical Review*, Durey, and *The Lancet* are all in Michael Durey, *The Return of the Plague: British Society and the Cholera, 1831–32* (Dublin: Gill & MacMillan, 1979), 7, 111, 111–12, 136.

The quote from the Indian Sanitary Commissioner is in Arnold, *Colonizing the Body*, 191.

The Italian delegate and the *Times of India* are quoted in Valeska Huber, "The Unification of the Globe by Disease? The International Sanitary Conferences on Cholera, 1851–1894," *Historical Journal* 49, no. 2 (2006): 464, 473.

Chapter 5: Tuberculosis

Marx and Engels are quoted in Helen Bynum, *Spitting Blood: The History of Tuberculosis* (Oxford: Oxford University Press, 2012), 112.

The Cummins quote is from S. Lyle Cummins, "Tuberculosis and the Empire," *British Journal of Tuberculosis* 31 (1937): 140–43, 141.

The Wilcocks quote is from Charles Wilcocks, "Presidential Address on Tuberculosis and Industry in Africa," *Royal Sanitary Institute* 73, no. 5 (1953): 481.

The Ransome quote is from Arthur J. Ransome, "Some Evidence Respecting Tubercular Infective Areas," *Transactions of the Epidemiological Society* 7 (1886–87): 124.

The Times quote is in David S. Barnes, "Historical Perspectives on the Etiology of Tuberculosis," *Microbes and Infection* 2, no. 4 (2000): 434.

The Long quote is in Esmond Long, "Artificial Pneumothorax in Tuberculosis," *American Journal of Nursing* 19, no. 4 (1919): 265, 268.

Public Health Commissioner of Bombay quoted in Niels Brimnes, "Languished Hopes" (unpublished manuscript in author's possession), 48.

The Wilcocks quote on lesions is in Charles Wilcocks, "Tuberculosis in the Natives of Tropical and Subtropical Regions," *Transactions of the Royal Society of Tropical Medicine and Hygiene*, 32, no. 6 (1939): 681.

The WHO quote on the largest mass action is in WHO, "Vaccination Against Tuberculosis, WHO Experts to Meet in Copenhagen," November 27, 1953, Press Release WHO/70, MOH 3/742, Kenya National Archives.

The WHO quote on possibilities is in Neil Brimnes, "Between Social, Cultural and Bacteriological Frames: Shifting Approaches to Tuberculosis in India c. 1920–1960," (unpublished manuscript in author's possession).

The McDermott quote on advances in biomedicine is in Walsh McDermott, "Tuberculosis at Home and Abroad," *Bulletin of the National Tuberculosis and Respiratory Disease Association* 54, no. 10 (1968): 11.

The Hecatomb quote is from J. Prignot and J. Sonnet, "AIDS, Tuberculosis, and Mycobacterioses," *Bulletin of the International Union against Tuberculosis and Lung Disease* 62, no. 4 (1987): 9.

The statement of the WHO and the International Union can be found in "HIV and Tuberculosis: Implications for TB Control Strategies and Agenda for Collaboration of AIDS and TB Programmes," WHO/TB/ CARG(4)/94.4, Archives of the International Union Against Tuberculosis and Lung Disease, Paris, France.

The Harries quote is in Anthony D. Harries et al., "The HIV-Associated Tuberculosis Epidemic—When Will We Act?" *The Lancet* 375 (2010): 1906.

Chapter 6: Influenza

The *British Medical Journal* quote is found in Susan Kingsley Kent, *The Influenza Pandemic of 1918-1919: A Brief History with Documents* (Boston: Bedford/St. Martin's, 2013), 64.

The quote from the Italian doctor is in Eugenia Tognotti, "Scientific Triumphalism and Learning From Facts: Bacteriology and the 'Spanish Flu' Challenge of 1918," *Social History of Medicine* 16, no. 1 (2003): 101.

For Sierra Leone being "upside down" see Don C. Ohadike, "Diffusion and Physiological Responses to the Influenza Pandemic of 1918–19 in Nigeria," *Social Science and Medicine* 32, no. 12 (1991): 1395.

The colonial official remarking on the Lobis is in David K. Patterson, "The Influenza Epidemic of 1918–19 in the Gold Coast," *Journal of African History* 24, no. 4 (1983): 491.

On Oakes's figure being "ludicrously low" see Niall P. A. S. Johnson and Juergen Mueller, "Updating the Accounts: Global Mortality of the 1918–1920 'Spanish' Influenza Pandemic," *Bulletin of the History of Medicine* 76, no. 1 (2002): 108.

The quote from the British agent regarding Tonga is in Sandra M. Tomkins, "The Influenza Epidemic of 1918–19 in Western Samoa," *Journal of Pacific History* 27, no. 2 (1992): 190. The goals of the commission are in Samoan Epidemic Commission, *Samoan Epidemic Commission (Report of), Presented to Both Houses of the General Assembly by Command of His Excellency* (Wellington, New Zealand: Government Printer, 1919), 7.

The quote on how we're still unable to predict a pandemic is from David M. Morens, Jeffery K. Taubenberger, Gregory K. Folkers, and Anthony S. Fauci, "Pandemic Influenza's 500th Anniversary," *Clinical Infectious Diseases* 51, no. 12 (2010): 1444.

The quote on the pandemic being a "point of departure" is in Kent, *Influenza Pandemic of 1918-1919*, 111.

The quote from the native commissioner and the Native Department in Rhodesia are in Terence Ranger, "The Influenza Pandemic in Southern Rhodesia: A Crisis of Comprehension," in David Arnold, ed., *Imperial Medicine and Indigenous Societies* (Manchester, UK: Manchester University Press, 1988), 177, 178.

Quotes regarding Bloemfontein, South Africa, are in Howard Phillips, "The Local State and Public Health Reform in South Africa: Bloemfontein and the Consequences of the Spanish 'Flu Epidemic of 1918,'" *Journal of Southern African Studies* 13, no. 2 (1987): 211, 218, 224.

Quotes from the *British Medical Journal*, the *Manchester Guardian*, and Newsholme are in Sandra M. Tomkins, "The Failure of Expertise: Public Health Policy in Britain during the 1918–19 Influenza Epidemic," *Social History of Medicine* 5, no. 3 (1992): 440, 444.

The quote from *The Times* comparing influenza to the Black Death is in Niall P. A. S. Johnson, "The Overshadowed Killer: Influenza in Britain, 1918–19," in *The Spanish Influenza of 1918-19: New Perspectives*, ed. Howard Phillips and David Killingray (New York: Routledge, 2003), 155.

"So vast was the catastrophe" from the *Times* is quoted in David Killingray, "A New 'Imperial Disease': The Influenza Pandemic of 1918-9 and Its Impact on the British Empire," *Caribbean Quarterly* 49, no. 4 (2003): 32.

Rosenau is quoted in Nancy K. Bristow, *American Pandemic: The Lost Worlds of the 1918 Influenza Epidemic* (New York: Oxford University Press, 2012), 159.

Chapter 7: HIV/AIDS

For the slow global response see Michael H. Merson, Jeffrey O'Malley, David Serwadda, and Chantawipa Apisuk, "The History and Challenge of HIV Prevention," *The Lancet* 372, no. 9637 (2008): 475–88.

Mahler is quoted in John Iliffe, *The African AIDS Epidemic* (Athens: Ohio University Press, 2006), 68.

Project SIDA's work was documented in Thomas C. Quinn, Jonathan M. Mann, James W. Curran, and Peter Piot, "AIDS in Africa: An Epidemiologic Paradigm," *Science* 234 (1986): 955–63.

The UNAIDS quote is in Joint United Nations Programme on HIV/AIDS, *UNAIDS: The First Ten Years* (2008), UNAIDS/07.20E/JC1262E, 7.

On the shift from the WHO to the World Bank see "Editorial: The World Bank's Cure for Donor Fatigue," *The Lancet* 342, no. 8863 (1993): 63.

The two articles from *The Lancet* are Elliot Marseille, Paul B. Hofmann, and James G. Kahn, "HIV Prevention before HAART in Sub-Saharan Africa," *The Lancet* 359, no. 9320 (2002): 1851–1856, 1851, and Andrew Creese, Katherine Floyd, Anita Alban, and Lorna Guinness, "Cost-Effectiveness of HIV/AIDS Interventions in Africa: A Systematic Review of the Evidence," *The Lancet* 359, no. 9318 (2002): 1638.

South Africa abrogating "patent rights" is in Messac and Prabhu, "Redefining the Possible," 122.

For Bush's remarks see George W. Bush, "Address before a Joint Session of the Congress on the State of the Union, January 28, 2003," in *Weekly Compilation of Presidential Documents* 39, no. 5 (2003), available at http://www.gpo.gov/fdsys/pkg/WCPD-2003-02-03/pdf/WCPD-2003-02-03.pdf.

Further reading

General

The most comprehensive overview of epidemic and pandemic disease (disease in general, really) is Kenneth Kiple, ed., *The Cambridge World History of Human Disease* (Cambridge, UK: Cambridge University Press, 1993). William McNeill's *Plagues and Peoples* (New York: Anchor, 1998; originally published in 1976) is a classic. Particularly useful for writing this book have been Mark Harrison, *Disease and the Modern World: 1500 to the Present Day* (Oxford: Polity, 2004); J. N. Hays, *The Burdens of Disease: Epidemics and Human Response in Western History*, 2nd ed. (New Brunswick, NJ: Rutgers University Press, 2009); and Roy Porter, *The Greatest Benefit to Mankind: A Medical History of Humanity* (New York: Norton, 1997). An excellent collection of essays, including a superb introduction on what historians might learn from epidemics and why they are so fascinated with them, is Terence Ranger and Paul Slack, eds., *Epidemics and Ideas: Essays on the Historical Perception of Pestilence* (Cambridge, UK: Cambridge University Press, 1992). An excellent discussion of the ways in which we might think about epidemics and pandemics historically is Charles E. Rosenberg, "What Is an Epidemic? AIDS in Historical Perspective," *Daedalus* 118, no. 2 (1989): 1–17. For a guide to the literature on epidemics and pandemics generally see Christian W. McMillen, "Epidemic Diseases and Their Effects on History," *Oxford Bibliographies Online*.

Chapter 1: Plague

The literature on plague is enormous—larger than any other pandemic historiography. Much of that literature is focused on the Black Death. However, for an excellent introduction that covers all plague pandemics see Paul Slack, *Plague: A Very Short Introduction* (New York: Oxford University Press, 2012). Slack's volume in the Very Short Introduction series has an excellent suggested readings list that is more comprehensive than what follows. A classic, only available in French, is Jean-Nöel Biraben, *Les Hommes et la Peste en France et Dans les Pays Europeens et Mediterraneens*, 2 vols. (Paris: Mouton, 1975).

For the first pandemic consult the essential Lester K. Little, ed., *Plague and the End of Antiquity: The Pandemic of 541-750* (Cambridge, UK: Cambridge University Press, 2007). Lawrence I. Conrad has studied the pandemic in the Middle East more thoroughly than anyone; see his "Epidemic Disease in Central Syria in the Late Sixth Century: Some New Insights from the Verse of Ḥassān ibn Thābit," *Byzantine and Greek Studies* 18, no. 1 (1994): 12–59, and "The Plague of Bilad al-Sham in Pre-Islamic Times," in *Proceedings of the Symposium on Bilad al-Sham during the Byzantine Period*, ed. Muhammad Adnan Bakhit (Amman: University of Jordan, 1996).

On the Black Death a worthwhile overview is John Kelly, *The Great Mortality: An Intimate History of the Black Death, the Most Devastating Plague of All Time* (New York: Harper, 2006). The most comprehensive history is Ole J. Benedictow, *The Black Death, 1346-1353: The Complete History* (Woodbridge, UK: Boydell, 2004). On the Middle East see Michael Dols, *The Black Death in the Middle East* (Princeton, NJ: Princeton University Press, 1977).

Beyond the Black Death there are many excellent histories. On the flourishing of medical writing on the plague see Samuel K. Cohn, *Cultures of Plague: Medical Thinking at the End of the Renaissance* (Oxford: Oxford University Press, 2010). The collection of essays edited by Vivian Nutton brings together many interdisciplinary perspectives on the plague: *Pestilential Complexities: Understanding Medieval Plague* (London: Wellcome Trust Centre for the History of Medicine, 2008). The plague's place in the Ottoman Empire is not as well understood as its role elsewhere. See Nukhet Varlik, *Plague and*

Pandemics

Empire in the Early Modern Mediterranean World: The Ottoman Experience, 1347–1600 (New York: Cambridge University Press, 2015), and Daniel Panzac, *La Peste dans l'Empire Ottoman, 1700–1850* (Louvain: Éditions Peeters, 1985). For the plague in early modern England see Paul Slack's indispensable *The Impact of Plague in Tudor and Stuart England* (London: Routledge & Kegan Paul, 1985). Carlo M. Cipolla's *Faith, Reason, and the Plague in Seventeenth Century Tuscany* (New York: Norton, 1979) is a model of historical writing.

The third pandemic has also benefited from much excellent historical writing. On the origins of the pandemic as it made its way through and out of China see Carol Benedict, *Bubonic Plague in Nineteenth-Century China* (Stanford, CA: Stanford University Press, 1996). For an overview of the pandemic in cities see Myron Echenberg, *Plague Ports: The Global Urban Impact of Bubonic Plague, 1894–1901* (New York: New York University Press, 2007). A good overview of the ways in which the global community tried to cope with plague, among other issues, is Mark Harrison, "Plague and the Global Economy," in his *Contagion: How Commerce Has Spread Disease* (New Haven, CT: Yale University Press, 2012), 174–210. The plague in India has been the subject of a number of excellent articles and chapters. See especially Rajnarayan Chandavarkar, "Plague Panic and Epidemic Politics in India, 1896–1914," in Ranger and Slack, *Epidemics and Ideas*, 203–40, and David Arnold, "Plague: Assault on the Body," in his *Colonizing the Body: State Medicine and Epidemic Disease in Nineteenth-Century India* (Berkeley: University of California Press, 1993), 200–239.

Chapter 2: Smallpox

Smallpox does not have nearly the same historiographical depth as the plague. There are, however, many excellent works that I have relied on. The only real overview is Donald R. Hopkins's *The Greatest Killer: Smallpox in History* (Chicago: University of Chicago Press, 2002). It is indispensable and covers the development of vaccination, for example, very well.

The literature on American Indians and disease generally is abundant. The debates over the population of the Americas in 1491 have gone on for decades. I have relied heavily on Elizabeth Fenn, *Pox Americana:*

The Great Smallpox Epidemic of 1775–82 (New York: Hill & Wang, 2001), and David S. Jones, *Rationalizing Epidemics: Meanings and Uses of American Indian Mortality since 1600* (Cambridge, MA: Harvard University Press, 2004). Paul Kelton has written two essential books that discuss smallpox: *Epidemics and Enslavement: Biological Catastrophe in the Native Southeast, 1492–1715* (Lincoln: University of Nebraska Press, 2007) and *Cherokee Medicine: An Indigenous Nation's Fight Against Smallpox, 1518–1824* (Norman: University of Oklahoma Press, 2015). James Daschuk's *Clearing the Plains: Disease, Politics, and the Loss of Aboriginal Life* (Regina, SK: University of Regina Press, 2013) does a superb job explaining how smallpox caused ethnogenesis on the Canadian plains and in the Great Lakes region. On bringing smallpox to the New World see Dauril Alden and Joseph C. Miller, "Out of Africa: The Slave Trade and the Transmission of Smallpox to Brazil, 1560–1831," *Journal of Interdisciplinary History* 18, no. 2 (1987): 195–224. Historians now generally reject the notion that American Indian susceptibility to disease was the sole cause of their demographic demise. Instead, they argue that population collapse was due to myriad factors such as warfare, competition over land, and malnutrition, among other things. See Catherine M. Cameron, Paul Kelton, and Alan C. Swedlund, eds., *Beyond Germs: Native Depopulation in the Americas* (Tucson: University of Arizona Press, 2015).

For vaccination's reception around the globe see the essays found in Sanjoy Bhattacharya and Niels Brimnes, eds., "Reassessing Smallpox Vaccination, 1789–1900," special issue, *Bulletin of the History of Medicine* 83, no. 1 (2009). Ann Jannetta's *The Vaccinators: Smallpox, Medical Knowledge, and the Opening of Japan* (Stanford, CA: Stanford University Press, 2007) and Brett L. Walker's "The Early Modern Japanese State and Ainu Vaccinations: Redefining the Body Politic 1799–1868," *Past and Present* 163 (1999): 121–60 are both excellent works on the connections between the history of state growth and infectious disease. For resisting smallpox vaccination see Nadja Durbach, "'They Might As Well Brand Us:' Working-Class Resistance to Compulsory Vaccination in Victorian England," *Social History of Medicine* 13, no. 1 (2000): 45–62. On this theme see Michael Willrich, *Pox: An American History* (New York: Penguin, 2011).

For smallpox in Europe see Hopkins, *Greatest Killer*, but also the chapters concerning smallpox in Peter Baldwin, *Contagion and the*

State in Europe, 1830–1930 (Cambridge, UK: Cambridge University Press, 1999). Also important is Ann. G. Carmichael and Arthur M Silverstein, "Smallpox in Europe before the Seventeenth Century: Virulent Killer or Benign Disease?" *Journal of the History of Medicine and Allied Sciences* 42, no. 2 (1987): 147–68.

William H. Schneider's overview "Smallpox in Africa during Colonial Rule," *Medical History* 53, no. 2 (2009): 193–277 is excellent.

The efforts to eradicate the disease are well covered in Sanjoy Bhattacharya, *Expunging Variola: The Control and Eradication of Smallpox in India, 1947–1977* (New Delhi: Orient Blackswan, 2006), and Nancy Leys Stepan, *Eradication: Ridding the World of Diseases Forever* (Ithaca, NY: Cornell University Press, 2011). The WHO chronicled its efforts in a massive and essential volume, now available electronically: Frank Fenner, Donald A. Henderson, Isao Arita, Zdeněk Ježek, and Ivan Danilovich Ladnyi, *Smallpox and Its Eradication* (Geneva: World Health Organization, 1988), available at http://apps.who.int/iris/bitstream/10665/39485/1/9241561106.pdf.

Chapter 3: Malaria

Randall Packard's *The Making of a Tropical Disease: A Short History of Malaria* (Baltimore: Johns Hopkins University Press, 2007) and James Webb's *Humanity's Burden: A Global History of Malaria* (New York: Cambridge University Press, 2009) are both essential reading, and I have based much of the chapter on these two books.

Malaria's arrival in and myriad effects on the New World is the subject of many books and articles. Among the best are Philip D. Curtin, "Disease Exchange Across the Tropical Atlantic," *History and Philosophy of the Life Sciences* 15, no. 3 (1993): 329–56; Mark Harrison, "'The Tender Frame of Man': Disease, Climate and Racial Difference in India and the West Indies, 1760–1860," *Bulletin of the History of Medicine* 70, no. 1 (1996): 69–93; and J. R. McNeill, *Mosquito Empires: Ecology and War in the Greater Caribbean, 1620–1914* (Cambridge, UK: Cambridge University Press, 2010).

On the ways in which malaria, migrant labor, and agriculture go hand in hand, see Alan Jeeves, "Migrant Workers and Epidemic Malaria on the South African Sugar Estates, 1906–1948," in Alan Jeeves and

Jonathan S. Crush, *White Farms, Black Labor: The State and Agrarian Change in Southern Africa, 1910–1950* (Pietermaritzburg, South Africa: University of Natal Press, 1997), 114–36. See also Randall M. Packard, "Maize, Cattle and Mosquitoes: The Political Economy of Malaria Epidemics in Colonial Swaziland," *Journal of African History* 25, no. 2 (1984): 189–212.

The effort to control malaria and the development of a variety of ways to do it is well told in Frank Snowden, *The Conquest of Malaria, Italy, 1900–1962* (New Haven, CT: Yale University Press, 2006), and Margaret Humphreys, *Malaria: Poverty, Race, and Public Health in the United States* (Baltimore: Johns Hopkins University Press, 2001). The difficulties associated with controlling malaria in Africa are the subject of James L. A. Webb, Jr., *The Long Struggle against Malaria in Tropical Africa* (Cambridge, UK: Cambridge University Press, 2014).

Nancy Leys Stepan's *Eradication: Ridding the World of Diseases Forever?* (Ithaca, NY: Cornell University Press, 2011) and Packard's *The Making of a Tropical Disease* are essential for understanding the impulse to eradicate generally and the Malaria Eradication Campaign specifically.

Chapter 4: Cholera

Two articles especially have had an enormous impact on the historiography of cholera and infectious disease generally. They are Asa Briggs, "Cholera and Society in the Nineteenth Century," *Past and Present* 19 (1961): 76–96, and Erwin H. Ackernecht, "Anticontagionism between 1821 and 1867," *Bulletin of the History of Medicine* 22 (1948): 562–93.

I have relied heavily on Christopher Hamlin's *Cholera: The Biography* (New York: Oxford University Press, 2009). It is wide-ranging and authoritative. Three excellent guides to cholera in Europe in the nineteenth century, especially the growth of the modern state and developments in medical theory, are Baldwin, *Contagion and the State*; Frank M. Snowden, *Naples in the Time of Cholera, 1884–1911* (Cambridge, UK: Cambridge University Press, 1995); and Richard J. Evans, *Death in Hamburg: Society and Politics in the Cholera Years, 1830–1910* (Oxford: Oxford University Press, 1987).

The growth of medical internationalism and cholera are best chronicled in William F. Bynum, "Policing Hearts of Darkness:

Aspects of the International Sanitary Conferences," *History and Philosophy of the Life Sciences* 15, no. 3 (1993): 421–34, and Valeska Huber, "The Unification of the Globe by Disease? The International Sanitary Conferences on Cholera, 1851–1894," *Historical Journal* 49, no. 2 (2006): 453–76.

Despite the overwrought title, Steven Johnson's *The Ghost Map: The Story of London's Most Terrifying Epidemic—and How It Changed Science, Cities, and the Modern World* (New York: Riverhead, 2006) is a compelling account of the work of John Snow and the changing ideas concerning disease transmission.

On cholera in India, David Arnold's *Colonizing the Body* is the place to start.

Myron Echenberg's *Africa in the Time of Cholera: A History of Pandemics from 1817 to the Present* (Cambridge, UK: Cambridge University Press, 2011) is essential. On the United States see Charles E. Rosenberg, *The Cholera Years: The United States in 1832, 1849, and 1866* (Chicago: University of Chicago Press, 1987; originally published in 1966).

Chapter 5: Tuberculosis

There are several overviews of TB. Helen Bynum's *Spitting Blood: A History of Tuberculosis* (Oxford: Oxford University Press, 2012) is the most recent and the one I turned to most frequently. Frank Ryan's *The Forgotten Plague: How the Battle against Tuberculosis Was Won—and Lost* (Boston: Little, Brown, 1994) and Thomas Dormandy's *The White Death: A History of Tuberculosis* (London: Hambledon, 1999) are also very valuable.

On TB's effect on medicine and society in a variety of different places I have relied on the following:

For England: Ann Hardy, *The Epidemic Streets: Infectious Disease and the Rise of Preventive Medicine, 1856–1900* (Oxford: Clarendon, 1993), and Linda Bryder, *Below the Magic Mountain: A Social History of Tuberculosis in Twentieth-Century Britain* (Oxford: Clarendon, 1988). For France: David S. Barnes, *The Making of a Social Disease: Tuberculosis in Nineteenth-Century France* (Berkeley: University of California Press, 1995). For the United States: Samuel K. Roberts, Jr.,

Infectious Fear: Politics, Disease, and the Health Effects of Segregation
(Chapel Hill: University of North Carolina Press, 2009); Mark
Caldwell, *The Last Crusade: The War on Consumption, 1862–1954*
(New York: Atheneum, 1988); and Sheila M. Rothman, *Living in the
Shadow of Death: Tuberculosis and the Social Experience of Illness in
American History* (New York: Basic Books, 1994). For South Africa:
Randall Packard, *White Plague, Black Labor: Tuberculosis and the
Political Economy of Health and Disease in South Africa* (Berkeley:
University of California Press, 1989).

For efforts to control TB internationally with antibiotics and the BCG
vaccine, as well as the TB/HIV pandemic and neoliberal thinking, see
my book *Discovering Tuberculosis: A Global History, 1900 to the
Present* (New Haven, CT: Yale University Press, 2015).

An excellent collection of essays on the contemporary TB pandemic is
Matthew Gandy and Alimuddin Zumla, eds., *Return of the White Plague:
Global Poverty and the "New" Tuberculosis* (London: Verso, 2003).

Chapter 6: Influenza

On influenza pandemics before 1918–1919 see K. David Patterson,
Pandemic Influenza, 1700–1900: A Study in Historical Methodology
(Totowa, NJ: Rowman & Littlefield, 1986).

The 1918–1919 pandemic has generated a lot of excellent historical
work. It has also spurred much biomedical work concerning the
origins of the pandemic as well as why it was so severe, among other
things. There are several overviews of the pandemic in the United
States; all are well worth reading: Alfred W. Crosby, *America's
Forgotten Pandemic: The Influenza of 1918*, 2nd ed. (Cambridge,
UK: Cambridge University Press, 1989), which covers regions
outside the United States as well; John M. Barry's *The Great
Influenza: The Epic Story of the Deadliest Plague in History* (New
York: Penguin, 2004) is especially well detailed and has much on
the history of virology; Nancy K. Bristol's *American Pandemic: The
Lost Worlds of the 1918 Influenza Epidemic* (New York: Oxford
University Press, 2012) does an excellent job chronicling what the
experience of influenza was like as well as discussing the hubris of
modern medicine.

The global pandemic, especially its effects in places like Samoa, Africa, Iran, India, and England, has also been the subject of superb histories. For an overview see the essays in Howard Phillips and David Killingray, eds., *The Spanish Influenza Pandemic of 1918–19: New Perspectives* (New York: Routledge, 2003). On India see I. D. Mills, "The 1918–1919 Influenza Pandemic: The Indian Experience," *Indian Economic and Social History Review* 23, no. 1 (1986): 1–40. For the pandemic's effects in Iran, Amir Afkhami's "Compromised Constitutions: The Iranian Experience with 1918 Influenza Pandemic," *Bulletin of the History of Medicine* 77, no. 2 (2003): 367–92 should be consulted. The pandemic had a devastating effect in the Pacific islands, especially in Western Samoa. Sandra Tomkins, "The Influenza Epidemic of 1918–19 in Western Samoa," *Journal of Pacific History* 27, no. 2 (1992): 181–97 tells the story in all its gruesome detail. The pandemic's wrath in Africa is the subject of a rich body of work; some is cited in the references. For a guide consult Matthew Heaton and Toyin Falola, "Global Explanations Versus Local Interpretations: The Historiography of the Influenza Pandemic of 1918–19 in Africa," *History in Africa* 33 (2006): 205–30.

The place of flu in American life, science, and public health policy is discussed in George Dehner, *Influenza: A Century of Science and Public Health Response* (Pittsburgh: University of Pittsburgh Press, 2012).

Mike Davis's *The Monster at our Door: The Global Threat of Avian Flu* (New York: Owl, 2005) is a good overview of the world's preparedness and the conditions that might give rise to a pandemic.

Among the most accessible articles in the biomedical literature are Jeffery K. Taubenberger, "The Origin and Virulence of the 1918 'Spanish' Influenza Virus," *Proceedings of the American Philosophical Society* 150, no. 1 (2006): 86–112, and J. K. Taubenberger, A. H. Reid, T. A. Janczewski, and T. G. Fanning, "Integrating Historical, Clinical and Molecular Genetic Data in Order to Explain the Origin and Virulence of the 1918 Spanish Influenza Virus," *Philosophical Transactions of the Royal Society of London* 356, no. 1416 (2001): 1829–39.

Chapter 7: HIV/AIDS

The AIDS literature is massive; not much of it is historical. For a general introduction to the disease Alan Whiteside's *HIV/AIDS: A Very*

Short Introduction is an excellent place to start. A solid historical overview can be found in Jonathan Engel, *The Epidemic: A Global History of AIDS* (New York: Smithsonian, 2006). To understand the pandemic in Africa see Helen Epstein, *The Invisible Cure: Africa, The West, and the Fight against AIDS* (New York: Farrar, Straus & Giroux, 2007), and John Iliffe, *The African AIDS Epidemic: A History* (Oxford: James Currey, 2006). While Jacques Pepin's *The Origins of AIDS* (Cambridge, UK: Cambridge University Press, 2011) is the best single volume explaining where AIDS likely came from and how it traveled.

The activist movement and the origins of citizen scientists—and much more—are the subject of Stephen Epstein, *Impure Science: AIDS, Activism, and the Politics of Knowledge* (Berkeley: University of California Press, 1996).

For a detailed look at how the United States and many countries in western Europe confronted AIDS, see Peter Baldwin, *Disease and Democracy: The Industrialized World Faces AIDS* (Berkeley: University of California Press, 2005).

The neglect of the pandemic can be found in Greg Behrman, *The Invisible People: How the U.S. Slept Through the Global AIDS Pandemic, the Greatest Humanitarian Catastrophe of Our Time* (New York: Free Press, 2004).

Paula A. Treichler's collection of essays *How to Have Theory in an Epidemic: Cultural Chronicles of AIDS* (Durham, NC: Duke University Press, 1999) is essential reading.

The role of neoliberalism and its transformation of the WHO, the World Bank, and AIDS policy is very important. To understand this relationship see Nitsan Chorev, *The World Health Organization Between North and South* (Ithaca, NY: Cornell University Press, 2012), and Luke Messac and Krishna Prabhu, "Redefining the Possible: The Global AIDS Response," in *Reimagining Global Health: An Introduction*, ed. Paul Farmer, Jim Yong Kim, Arthur Kleinman, and Mathew Basilico (Berkeley: University of California Press, 2013),

111–32. This essay also covers the changes in thinking regarding access to drugs and their costs as well as AIDS activism.

For the myriad ways in which AIDS has changed global health see Allan M. Brandt, "How AIDS Invented Global Health," *New England Journal of Medicine* 368, no. 23 (2013): 2149–52.

"牛津通识读本"已出书目

德国文学	儿童心理学	电影
戏剧	时装	俄罗斯文学
腐败	现代拉丁美洲文学	古典文学
医事法	卢梭	大数据
癌症	隐私	洛克
植物	电影音乐	幸福
法语文学	抑郁症	免疫系统
微观经济学	传染病	银行学
湖泊	希腊化时代	景观设计学
拜占庭	知识	神圣罗马帝国
司法心理学	环境伦理学	大流行病